THE CHIROPRACTIC PROFESSION

Its Education, Practice, Research and Future Directions

David A. Chapman-Smith LLB (Hons), PCE, FICC (Hon)
Secretary-General, World Federation of Chiropractic
Editor, The Chiropractic Report

Foreword by
Wayne B. Jonas MD
Director, Office of Alternative Medicine, National Institutes of Health (1995–1998)

NCMIC Group Inc.
West Des Moines, Iowa

For Lloyd, Leo and Lou, and for Sira.

Design, composition and printing: Harmony Printing Limited, Toronto, Canada
Project administration: Foundation for Chiropractic Education and Research

To purchase additional copies of this book call 1-877-291-7312 or fax orders to (515) 282-3347.

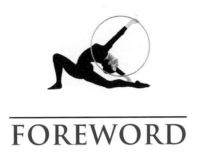

FOREWORD

If you had told me 20 years ago that a time would come when chiropractors and physicians would be working together in common clinics, when they would collaborate on chiropractic research funded by the federal government, and when chiropractic services would be recommended by medical and national organizations, I would have said you were crazy. Since this is all now happening, it shows how mistaken I—as a physician—would have been.

Still, when I was asked to write the foreword to a book for the public that a chiropractic publisher, the NCMIC Group, was going to produce, I was skeptical. How could a book from a source that was obviously pro-chiropractic provide a balanced view of the profession for the public? Again, my judgement was wrong. This book is a well-balanced, clear and detailed description of the chiropractic profession today.

Deep prejudice is hard to change. I began medical school right after the case of *Wilk* vs. *the American Medical Association* was filed. In that case, a federal court found my profession guilty of a prolonged and systematic attempt to completely undermine the profession of chiropractic, often using highly dishonest methods. Paradoxically, I found that the climate at my medical school was even more distrustful of chiropractors after the *Wilk* case. For many physicians, chiropractors were simply "quacks" not to be trusted, and they communicated this to their patients—often, interestingly, not knowing that many of these same patients were also seeing chiropractors. The cognitive dissonance such prejudice produced was considerable, but I still kept my distance from chiropractors. Referral to a chiropractor was simply not in my repertoire of care.

As director of the Office of Alternative Medicine (OAM) at the National Institutes of Health from the years 1995–1998, I began to work with chiropractors in developing research on the effects of manipulation and chiropractic care. I invited chiropractors to sit on the OAM Advisory Council and worked with the profession to establish a consortial research center for chiropractic research. The sophistication, professionalism, expertise and interest in science that I saw impressed me.

Gradually, my prejudice was softened. I visited a chiropractor for some neck pain, and then found a referral network of good chiropractors in my area for my patients with low-back pain and musculoskeletal problems. I have seen at all levels the truth of the statement by the Agency for Health Care Policy and Research report that "chiropractic has undergone a remarkable transformation."[1] So have I.

Those who will take the time to read this book are likely to find their attitudes—in favor or against—will also be transformed to a more realistic and balanced view. Unlike any other book, and after the many changes in recent years, it provides a concise and informative review of all relevant information on the chiropractic profession in one volume—including information on education, practice, research, origins and future directions.

Is chiropractic safe? The answer is yes. Only 1.5 serious adverse events per million manipulations occur. This is safer than many conventional therapies for the same problems. Is it completely safe? The answer is no. Adverse effects do occur and well-developed guidelines exist that should be followed to minimize the risks.

Is chiropractic effective? For certain types of low-back pain, headache and other musculoskeletal problems the answer is yes. For other problems the answer is we don't know yet—more high quality research is necessary before we can say yes or no.

Does chiropractic save money? Most studies, but not all, show that it does save money compared to conventional treatment. However this may be more an indictment of the high cost and poor effectiveness of many conventional treatments for back pain than confirmation of the optimal value of chiropractic.

Are patients who visit chiropractors satisfied? The answer is an overwhelming yes. Most studies, show that 80–90% of patients are satisfied with their care from a chiropractor—more satisfied than with their conventional physician.

Is there a science behind chiropractic? The answer is yes for some treatments and no for others, but the amount of science is increasing. This book summarizes much of that research showing that spinal manipulation can produce significant neurological and physiological effects. In addition, there are controlled trials and guidelines based on quality clinical research. Figure 2, in Chapter 8 (pages 112–113) provides a sophisticated summary of the evidence for chiropractic and medical management of back pain. Would that we had such evaluations for all conditions treated in mainstream medicine.

Are chiropractors qualified? For their legal and professional scope of practice the answer is yes. In their major area of practice, the evaluation and treatment of musculoskeletal problems, chiropractors have better training and experience than conventional physicians do. They have less training in medical management of other conditions, however.

Can you get chiropractic care? Access and availability, previously limited and paid for out of pocket, is now increasingly available and reimbursed by employers and insurance companies.

All is not rosy in chiropractic, however, and this book often points this out. If you visit a chiropractor you may need to do so nearly a dozen times and sometimes several times a week before benefit sets in. This may be inconvenient or costly for many people. Some chiropractors (estimated to be about 4–5% of the profession) still go beyond their area of expertise in treating diseases for which they are not qualified, and in selling dietary supplements and products that are unproven and possibly harmful or dangerous. You must be wary of this.

As in conventional medicine, much of what chiropractors do has not been proven by clinical trials, so there is considerably uncertainty, subjectivity and room for variation in practice. Whether you are a prospective patient or a physician considering referral of patients this book will help you understand the basics of what chiropractors can and cannot do. Caution and common sense should always be used when making individual treatment choices.

Chiropractic "has emerged from the periphery of the health care system and is playing a increasingly important role in discussion of health care policy."[1] After a century of both suppression and isolationism, the chiropractic profession is assuming its valuable and appropriate role in the health care system in this country and around the world. As this happens, the professional battles of the past will fade and the patient at last will be the true winner.

Wayne B. Jonas, M.D.
Uniformed Services University of the Health Sciences Bethesda, Maryland. Director (1995–1998) Office of Alternative Medicine, National Institutes of Health

1 Chiropractic in the United States, training, practice and research. Cherkin DC, Mootz RD. eds. Publication No. 98-N002. U.S. Department of Health and Human Services, 1997.

TABLE OF CONTENTS

ACKNOWLEDGMENTS

A book such as this is the cumulative product of the efforts of many people. It is not possible to acknowledge all the help I have received. I must begin with thanks to the clinicians, educationalists and researchers in the chiropractic profession who gave me this tale to tell.

Special thanks are due to Anthony Rosner, PhD, Director of Education and Research, Foundation for Chiropractic Education and Research and Louis Sportelli, DC, President, NCMIC Group. They shepherded this project and led the team of reviewers, other members of which were Sira Borges, DC MD, John DeMatte IV, DC, Peter Dixon, DC, Robert Haig, DC, Deborah Kopansky-Giles, DC, Sil Mior, DC, Howard Vernon, DC, and Susan Wakefield. My thanks to them.

Many people interrupted busy schedules to render assistance with illustrations, and special thanks are due to Janet Blanchard-Conn at the Ontario Chiropractic Association, Satvinder Jhaj at the World Federation of Chiropractic, Donald Petersen, Jr. at Dynamic Chiropractic and Glenda Weise at Palmer College of Chiropractic. Finally I owe a great debt of thanks to Serena Smith for preparation of the manuscript,

Robin Merrifield for copy editing, and Ken Slater at Harmony Printing for book design and composition.

This book has accompanied me on my travels during the past year and was written in Brazil, Canada, Switzerland and the United States, all countries in which chiropractic education, practice and research are now flourishing. In it I endeavor to describe the state of the profession as it enters the year 2000. Although its integration into core health services is not yet complete, the chiropractic profession has made more impressive progress than many people appreciate. As a result this is perhaps a useful time to gather current information on the profession and place it in one volume.

I am most fortunate that my vague plans to undertake this work were crystallized by a proposal and grant from the NCMIC Group Inc. My goal has been to write a book that is suitable for both the public and other health care professionals, and which answers all of the questions you are likely to have about the chiropractic profession. You will be the judge of whether or not I have succeeded.

David Chapman-Smith
September 1999

SUMMARY FACTS ON CHIROPRACTIC

1. **Definition:** Chiropractic is a health profession concerned with the diagnosis, treatment and prevention of disorders of the musculoskeletal system, and the effects of these disorders on the nervous system and general health. There is an emphasis on manual treatments, including spinal manipulation.

   The word *chiropractic*, from the Greek words *praxis* and *cheir*, means practice or treatment by hand. Like the word *pharmaceutical* it is used both as an adjective (e.g. chiropractic profession) and as a noun (e.g. as in the definition above).

2. **Origin and Professional Organization:** The profession was founded in the U.S. in 1895 and is now established in over 70 countries. National associations of chiropractors from these countries are members of a World Federation of Chiropractic, based in Toronto, Canada, which is in official relations with the World Health Organization. There are approximately 65,000 doctors of chiropractic in the U.S., 6,000 in Canada and 90,000 internationally. (*For further details, see Chapter 3*).

3. **Education and Licensure:** In North America there is a minimum of six years full time university-level education, which includes two years of university credits in qualifying subjects and then a four year undergraduate program at chiropractic college. This is followed by national and state/provincial licensing board examinations. Postgraduate specialties include chiropractic sciences, neurology, nutrition, orthopedics, radiology, rehabilitation and sports chiropractic. (*See Chapter 4.*)

   Internationally, common standards of education have been achieved through a network of accrediting agencies that began with the U.S. Council on Chiropractic Education (CCE), recognized by the U.S. Office of Education since 1974. There are chiropractic colleges in Australia (2), Brazil, Canada (2), Denmark, France, Italy, Japan, Korea, New Zealand, South Africa, Sweden, the United Kingdom (4) and the United States (16). In most countries these colleges are now in the public university system. (*See Chapter 4.*)

4. **Licensing Laws:** The practice of chiropractic is now recognized and regulated by law in many countries in all world regions. Common features of all licensing laws are primary care (i.e. the right of a patient to consult a chiropractor directly), and the right and duty to perform a diagnosis. Diagnosis includes the right to use x-ray and other diagnostic imaging and tests. (*See Chapter 3.*)

5. **Title:** The professional titles most commonly approved by law in the U.S. states and Canadian provinces are *chiropractor* and *doctor of chiropractic*. Many U.S. states also approve the title *chiropractic physician*. In these states the title *physician* is given to chiropractic, medical and osteopathic doctors in recognition of their competence and duty to perform a diagnosis.

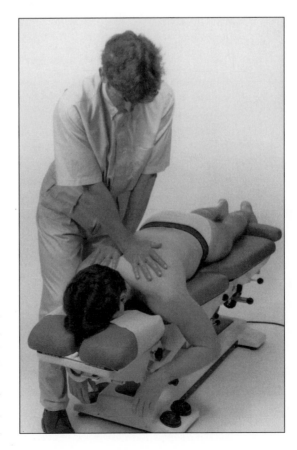

6. **Practice:** The chiropractic profession emphasizes the natural power of the body to heal itself (homeostasis) and therefore chiropractic practice does not include the use of drugs or surgery. Patients requiring these interventions are referred for medical care. Chiropractors use natural or non-invasive treatment approaches including manual treatments, physical therapy modalities, exercise programs, nutritional advice, orthotics, lifestyle modification and other patient education. (*See Chapters 5 and 6.*) There is an emphasis on joint manipulation, for which the traditional chiropractic term is joint adjustment, because of its proven effectiveness. (*See Chapter 7.*)

Surveys in Australia, Europe and North America report that approximately 95% of chiropractic patients have musculoskeletal pain conditions (e.g. back pain, neck pain, headache, pain in the shoulder, arms or legs) as their main complaint. Research and research-based practice guidelines from various multidisciplinary expert panels in the 1990s have endorsed chiropractic management by recommending spinal manipulation, over-the-counter pain medication, exercise and early return to activities as the most effective and cost-effective management for most patients with back pain, neck pain and tension-type headache. (*On headache/neck pain see Chapter 6, on back pain see Chapter 8.*)

The other 5% of chiropractic practice involves patients with a wide variety of conditions that are caused, aggravated or mimicked by restricted range of movement in the spinal vertebrae and muscles, termed spinal dysfunction or subluxation, and the pain and other reflex effects of this expressed through the nervous system. Such conditions include dysmenorrhea, asthma and other respiratory dysfunctions, colic, constipation and other digestive dysfunctions. (*See Chapters 5 and 6.*)

For various reasons, including improved chiropractic education and research during the past 20 years and the expectations—indeed the demands—of patients, much of the former conflict between the chiropractic and medical professions has been replaced by mutual respect and cooperation. Interdisciplinary practice is now common, with chiropractic and medical doctors, physical therapists and others working as partners or referring patients as necessary in general practice, occupational health, automobile accident and other rehabilitation centers and sports medicine teams. (*See Chapters 2 and 9.*)

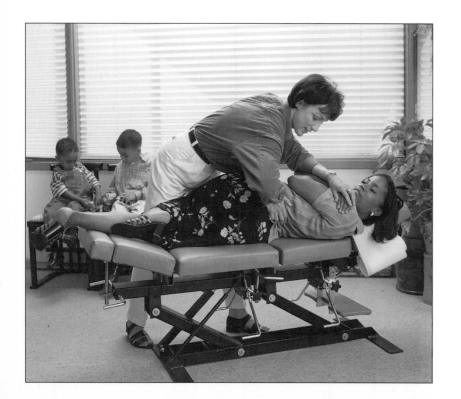

For illustrations of the main components of the neuromusculoskeletal system, diagrams giving a basic review of:
- *the skeleton,*
- *the pelvis and spine,*
- *associated nerves, muscles and ligaments,*

see Appendix 1 on page 155.

CHAPTER 1

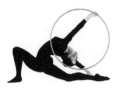

INTRODUCTION

"Spinal manipulation and the profession most closely associated with its use, chiropractic, have gained a legitimacy within the United States health care system that until very recently seemed unimaginable.

"In the past several decades, chiropractic has undergone a remarkable transformation. Labeled an 'unscientific cult' by organized medicine as little as 20 years ago chiropractic is now recognized as the principal source of one of the few treatments recommended by national evidence-based guidelines for the treatment of low-back pain, spinal manipulation. In the areas of training, practice, and research, chiropractic has emerged from the periphery of the health care system and is playing an increasingly important role in discussions of health care policy."

AHCPR Research Report, U.S. Department of Health and Human Services, 1997.[1]

This is how Daniel Cherkin, PhD, Senior Scientific Investigator, Group Health Cooperative of Puget Sound, Seattle, Washington, and Robert Mootz, DC, Associate Medical Director for Chiropractic, Department of Labor and Industries, Olympia, Washington, introduced a recent U.S. government-funded report for policy makers and health professionals titled *Chiropractic in the United States: Training, Practice and Research*. The report was prepared because other sources of information were "widely scattered, often biased and . . . often out of date."

The goal of this book is to provide a comprehensive overview of the chiropractic profession in a format and language suitable not only for health professionals but also for the general reader—patients, insurers, consumer advocates, journalists and anyone else who may be interested. From the index or table of contents you will see that there is comment on:

- History—including the reasons why there have been conflicts between chiropractors and physicians, with faults on both sides, and why this has now been replaced with widespread cooperation and understanding.

- Education—many people will be surprised to learn that there is a minimum of six years full-time university-level education, followed by licensing exams, before a person qualifies to practice as a chiropractor in the United States. There are similar requirements in the many other countries where chiropractic practice is now regulated by law.

- Chiropractic scope of practice—what chiropractors treat, how and why.

- Research and literature.

- Many other present developments—it may surprise you to learn that chiropractic and medical doctors often now practice together, that today there is as much scientific evidence supporting chiropractic manipulation for back pain as any other treatment, that a recent survey at a large California health maintenance organization (HMO) showed that a clear majority of primary care

The goal of this book is to provide a comprehensive overview of the chiropractic profession in language suitable not only for health professionals but also for the general reader.

physicians (55%) and patients (61%) wanted to have chiropractic services available at the HMO,[2] and that internationally many medical doctors are now enrolling at chiropractic colleges to re-qualify as chiropractors.

A. Sources and Quality of Evidence

The main goal of this introduction, written by an attorney, is to have you think about the various different sources of evidence on the chiropractic profession—how informed, biased or reliable they may be, and how much you should believe each of them.

What do you really know about the chiropractic profession? How reliable and accurate are your sources of information? How do you reconcile the conflicting good and bad news stories you still hear?

Health care is a very personal matter. But health care services, like automobiles, are also consumer items in a very competitive marketplace. Back pain and headache, the two conditions for which adults most frequently seek health care services, are each multi-billion dollar markets annually. Chiropractors, medical doctors, pharmaceutical companies and many other health professionals are competitors in that market which, until recently, was completely dominated by the medical profession.

Think of it this way: If you are planning to buy a new car, say a Toyota Camry, you know that you are going to get differing opinions from a Toyota salesperson, a Ford salesperson, satisfied and dissatisfied Camry owners, bogus customer survey research or vehicle performance ratings from a corporation established as a marketing device by Toyota or one of its competitors, properly designed market surveys from an independent institute endorsed by all major automobile manufacturers and other sources. Questions of expertise and conscious and unconscious bias arise—questions that are familiar to every litigation attorney but are often not so clearly understood by others.

If you are thinking of consulting—or, in market language, buying the services of—a health care professional because you suddenly have disabling back pain, who will give you the most reliable opinion on the best first approaches to diagnosis and treatment? Say, for argument's sake, you are thinking of consulting a chiropractor as a first option. You can expect very different information and opinions from:

- A chiropractic doctor (the Toyota sales rep)
- A medical doctor (the Ford sales rep)
- The national chiropractic association (Toyota Inc)
- The national medical association (Ford Motors Inc)
- A consumer advocate or organization (may be bogus or real—where does the advice, expertise or funding come from?)
- Chiropractic experts funded by the chiropractic profession (could be accurate, but suspect a bias in favor)
- Medical experts funded by the medical profession (could be accurate, suspect a bias against)
- A multidisciplinary team of researchers (could be good, but what is their experience, reputation and independence—see discussion below on scientific evidence)
- A multidisciplinary panel of experts—e.g. orthopedists, neurologists, chiropractors, physical medicine specialists, physical therapists, family physicians—selected and funded by a government agency (beginning to sound much more reliable)
- A judicial inquiry (if the witnesses include chiropractic and medical experts, whose views are tested by cross-examination, and the judge or commission is neutral and respected, there is finally some guarantee of independence and truth)

Evidence and opinions from all of these sources exist. Even the above list, which is quite long, represents a simplification. There are subcategories—for example a medical doctor may or may not have knowledge of chiropractic education and practice, referral relationships with a chiropractor where appropriate, an ax to grind, an active role in a trade medical association, an interest in a competing physical rehab facility, etc. In short he or she may be an excellent or an unreliable source of information. It is time to briefly illustrate these problems:

- In 1993–1994 government-sponsored interdisciplinary panels of experts in the U.S. and the U.K. reviewed the scientific literature on the management of adults with low-back pain. These experts then published clinical practice guidelines supporting spinal manipulation as a first line approach to the management of most patients with back pain.[3,4] However in May 1995 the American Medical Association (AMA), calling itself "the nation's most trusted health care authority" and expressly claiming to be providing "a reliable source of information" published the *AMA Pocket Guide to Back Pain*,[5] which was inconsistent with the guidelines in several major respects. One was that it made no mention at all of spinal manipulation, manual therapy or chiropractic treatment. It is fair to conclude that this was because the AMA wanted to support the treatments given by its members and medical doctors are not trained in and do not provide manipulation.

- As a second example let us look at two individuals who are long-term critics of chiropractors and who present themselves as unbiased consumer advocates, William Jarvis, PhD, Professor of Health Promotion and Education, Loma Linda University, California and President, National Council Against Health Fraud Inc, and Murray Katz, MD, a physician from Montreal, Quebec.

Dr. Jarvis, who presents evidence internationally against the chiropractic profession and has been a source of many negative articles on chiropractic over the past 20 years, writes in a 1995 foreword to a book titled *Chiropractic: The Victim's Perspective*, "chiropractic has still not made a single noteworthy contribution to the scientific knowledge of health care." In their education chiropractic students only learn bogus or "conversational" medicine which "enables them to speak as if they know about disease and healing processes and *creates the illusion that they understand medical science.*"[6] (Emphasis added)

Chiropractic education is dealt with in a later chapter in this book—you will see there that independent government and medical investigations have concluded that chiropractic education, far from being an "illusion" of understanding, is actually now the equal of medical education in anatomy, physiology and all the basic sciences (*Chapter 4*). To further illustrate Dr. Jarvis' bias and why his views on the chiropractic profession are questionable, let us look at his claim that the profession has "not made a single noteworthy contribution" to science. Many noteworthy scientific discoveries from the chiropractic profession include, for example, those of:

1. David Cassidy, DC, PhD, Canada—on the anatomy of the sacroiliac (SI) joint from embryonic life until old age,[7] and the prevalence of low-back pain and SI joint dysfunction in school children.[8]

   For diagrams illustrating relevant anatomy—the skeleton, the spine and pelvis including the SI joints, and associated nerves, muscles and ligaments, see Appendix 1 on page 155.

2. Lynton Giles, DC, PhD, Australia—on the anatomy of spinal facet joints in the low-back and the presence and nature of connec-

. . . the major scientific discovery of the chiropractic profession has been the value of skilled manipulation in the treatment of patients with many common and disabling conditions of low-back and neck pain.

   tive tissue tags that are often trapped in these joints.[9]

3. Gregory Cramer, DC, PhD and Barclay Bakkum, DC, PhD, United States—on the anatomy of the intervertebral foramen (IVF), the space between adjacent vertebrae through which the spinal nerves exit from the spinal cord—both the IVFs exact dimensions, measured by computer tomography and MRI, and transforaminal ligaments.[10]

4. Barry Mitchell, PhD and Kim Humphries, DC, PhD, United Kingdom—on the anatomy of the ligamentum nuchæ, a posterior ligament that stabilizes the upper cervical spine—specifically discovery of new attachments between this ligament and the skull and dura that provide a new anatomical basis for cervical spine or tension-type headache.[11]

5. Niels Nilsson, DC, MD, PhD, Denmark—on the frequency or prevalence of headache caused by joint and muscle tension in the neck (cervicogenic headache) and the effectiveness of treatment by chiropractic manipulation.[12,13] (Dr. Nilsson has shown that this type of headache, largely unrecognized by the medical profession until 1988, is as common as migraine [for which it is frequently misdiagnosed] and is more effectively treated by chiropractic manipulation than standard medical management. Surely this represents a noteworthy contribution to the scientific knowledge of health care.)

6. Generally, and most importantly from the public's perspective, the major scientific discovery or contribution of the chiropractic profession has been the value of skilled manipulation in the treatment of patients with many common and disabling conditions of low-back and neck pain. Spinal manipulation, once rejected by medical authorities, is now regarded as a first line approach to treatment.[3,4,14] Medical and physical therapy researchers have contributed to the body of knowledge. However no one can reasonably question the view that

"We have no idea whether the people joining (the Orthopractic Society) are good or bad manipulators and quite frankly we don't care."

the chiropractic profession has led education, practice and research in this field.

Most of these discoveries, including the scientific acceptance of spinal manipulation for most back pain patients, were published and apparent when Dr. Jarvis wrote his dismissive comments. Although he has a doctorate, a university position, communicates well and claims independence and knowledge of the chiropractic profession, can he be regarded as a reliable source of information?

The same question may be asked of Stephen Barrett, MD, a retired psychiatrist from Pennsylvania who has worked through the U.S. Con-

sumer's Union, and Murray Katz, MD, a physician from Montreal who has worked through the Consumer's Association of Canada. Both claim to be consumer advocates but, like Jarvis, have waged an emotional campaign against the chiropractic profession for over 20 years. The chiropractic profession remains perplexed as to why they have such ready access to and credibility with the media. In print and in person they display obvious bias.

In recent years Dr. Katz has even endeavored to create a new medically controlled profession called *orthopractic* to replace chiropractors in the health care system in the U.S. and Canada, telling the public this is necessary for reasons of competence and safety but telling medical audiences that it is for political reasons. Writing in the *Medical Post* he says this of the new specialty he wants to create to replace chiropractic:

"Orthopractic means to provide manual therapy in a safe, scientific and responsible manner."[15]

Two weeks later, speaking about orthopractic behind closed doors to the Ontario Medical Association he says:

"I am going to be talking about politics . . . we are not talking about clinical competence, not talking about science. . . . The point is the political reality that there are 60,000 chiropractors treating millions of people by manipulation.

"The name *orthopractic* was meant to mimic chiropractic. . . . We have no idea whether the people joining (the Orthopractic Society) are good or bad manipulators and quite frankly we don't care. . . . Orthopractic can now solve largely political problems, we are asking government to fund orthopractic only."[16]

Such contradictions of purpose raise serious questions of credibility. Are these the comments of a consumer advocate, someone concerned about quality care and the rights of patients? If the Consumers' Association of Canada gets its advice on chiropractic from Dr. Katz what weight should be given to its views—even if it is a consumers' association and does good work in other areas?

When Dr. Katz was subject to cross-examination on his views of chiropractic before a Commission of Inquiry in New Zealand in the late 1970s, the Commission had similar concern about his credibility. The Commission was "abundantly satisfied that it would be quite unsafe to rely on (Dr. Katz's) opinions or on any of his evidence on matters of fact" with respect to chiropractic.[17]

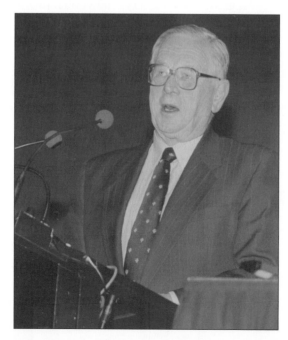

The Commission is "abundantly satisfied that it would be quite unsafe to rely on Dr. Katz's opinions or on any of his evidence on matters of fact (with respect to chiropractic)." Judge B. Donald Inglis, who was Chairman of the New Zealand Commission of Inquiry into Chiropractic, is seen here addressing the World Chiropractic Congress in Auckland, May 1999.

So, it is important to consider the background and reliability of information you hear about the chiropractic profession.

Is This Book Biased?

Because of these strong comments about critics of the chiropractic profession you may well be asking—quite rightly—how reliable is this book? It was commissioned by the NCMIC Group Inc., a U.S. chiropractic organization, and written by an attorney who represents the chiropractic profession. Continue to ask that question as you read. Presume some bias in favor of chiropractic, and check to see that important facts and conclusions are supported by reference to published research and other documents. Keep asking whether the sources and commentaries seem reliable. Place extra weight on independent and interdisciplinary evidence.

B. Levels of Scientific Evidence

Here are a few introductory comments to help you understand the rapidly changing world of scientific evidence. There is actually much less good scientific evidence for health care interventions than you might think—only about 15% of medical interventions are supported by valid scientific evidence.[18] Until fairly recently it was presumed that a randomized controlled trial published in a peer-reviewed journal (a scientific journal in which all draft articles are submitted anonymously to other researchers from that field for review and amendment before they are accepted for publication) was automatically good and sufficient evidence of whether a treatment worked or not. Today the health sciences community requires considerably more than that—two or more high quality trials and ideally an expert or systematic review based on several such trials.

Here are some different levels of evidence, from the weakest to the strongest in scientific terms.

1. **Case Study**. This is a report on one or more individual cases and merely represents the starting point for further serious research.

2. **A Retrospective Study**. This is done after treatment was given. Sometimes there is contact between the patient and researcher (case control study) and sometimes, as in studies reviewing file data only, there is not (observational study). This form of research is scientifically weak because many factors in diagnosis, treatment and recording of results are uncontrolled.

3. **A Prospective Study**. As the name indicates this study is designed prospectively or before treatment is given. With sound planning and design all important factors can be controlled and such studies may have considerable validity. The prospective study is standard research with a consecutive series of patients in a clinical setting. Its main limitations are:

   - There is no second comparative control group of patients. Therefore there is no way of knowing whether the patients, if they improve, would have improved anyway—even without the treatment. (In some circumstances this criticism may carry little weight. See, for example, the work of Kirkaldy-Willis and Cassidy with chiropractic treatment of a Canadian hospital population of patients with chronic low-back pain.[19] Given that these patients had been disabled for many years, the variety of prior treatments, the caliber of the researchers, the thoroughness of the design and the strong results achieved, this descriptive study is probably of equal scientific weight to any controlled trial yet performed for chronic pain patients.)

   - The patients have usually chosen the form of treatment themselves, or in other words are self-selected. This introduces an element of bias or unreliability. In a full trial an administrator randomly assigns them to one of the two or more treatment groups.

4. **Randomized Controlled Trial (RCT)**. The RCT or double-blind clinical trial is the most scientific method of testing the effectiveness of any health care treatment. However, trials performed vary considerably as to design and validity. The classical RCT tests the effectiveness of a defined treatment by giving it to one group of patients while a second comparable group receives a sham or placebo treatment. Adding another group with a second treatment allows the trial to show comparative effectiveness as well. For practical reasons, including the welfare of patients with serious disorders, there may be no sham or control treatment group, just different treatment groups—as for example in a comparison of medical and surgical treat-

ment for patients with acute angina. Other features of an RCT are:

a) Randomization. Patients meeting the eligibility criteria for entrance to the trial are randomly assigned to the trial groups. They, and those performing the trial, cannot choose the treatment received.

b) Double-blindness. Neither the patient nor those on the research team measuring results know which treatment was received, the real one or a sham one. Both are blind—the trial is double-blinded. The aim of this and other design features is to rule out all chance effects (eliminate bias) leaving only the effects of the therapy under trial.

Table 1 **Evidence Rating Systems Used in National Guidelines for Clinical Practice**

U.S. AHCPR RATING SYSTEM [1]

Used to rate or define levels of scientific evidence assessed by experts to support clinical guideline statements.

A. Strong research-based evidence (multiple relevant and high-quality scientific studies).

B. Moderate research-based evidence (one relevant, high-quality scientific study or multiple adequate scientific studies*).

C. Limited research-based evidence (at least one adequate scientific study* in patients with low-back pain).

D. Panel interpretation of information that did **not** meet inclusion criteria as research-based evidence.

*Met minimal formal criteria for scientific methodology and relevance to population and specific method addressed in guideline statement.

U.K. ROYAL COLLEGE OF GENERAL PRACTITIONERS RATING SYSTEM [2]

The evidence is weighted as follows:

◆◆◆   Generally consistent findings in a majority of acceptable studies

◆◆   Either based on a single acceptable study, or a weak or inconsistent finding in some of multiple acceptable studies.

◆   Limited scientific evidence, which does not meet all the criteria of 'acceptable' studies

---

1 Bigos S, Bowyer O, Braen G, et al. Acute low-back problems in adults. Clinical practice guideline No.14. Rockville, Maryland: Agency for Health Care Policy and Research, Public Health Service, U.S. Department of Health and Human Services, 1994; AHCPR Publication No. 95-0642.

2 Waddell G, Feder G, et al. Low-back pain evidence review. London, England: Royal College of General Practitioners, 1996.

C. The Purposes of Clinical Guidelines and Evidence Rating Systems

The problems with insisting upon strong scientific evidence (several RCTs assessed for value in a systematic review) are that:

- Few health care treatments have this level of scientific evidence, a problem that will not be resolved soon because of the time and cost involved.

- It ignores over 90% of the evidence, from clinical experience and case studies to prospective studies and pilot trials.

These problems are now widely recognized in the health sciences world and this has led to two important developments during the past 10 years:

1. **Development of clinical guidelines**. This is a formal process in which a representative panel of experts combines two sources of knowledge—the published research and clinical experience—and provides guidelines to health professionals on how best to manage patients with a given complaint. For back pain, for example, in the U.S. there are now chiropractic guidelines[20] and government-sponsored interdisciplinary guidelines[3] for management.

2. **Evidence rating systems**. This is a system of rating the level of reliability of the evidence. In other words one can and should place some weight on various levels of evidence, but only where a rating system is used to explain the level of evidence relied upon. Table 1 gives the rating systems used in the 1994 U.S. and the 1996 U.K. interdisciplinary back pain guidelines for all health professionals treating patients with back pain. Similar rating systems have been used in chiropractic guidelines.

If all of these comments on scientific evidence seem a little complicated. don't be concerned—you can take heart from the fact that only a small number of health professionals understand these things well. Most of those who understand are epidemiologists—medical doctors and others, including chiropractors, who have completed masters and doctorate degrees giving them specialized training in research methods. World-renowned epidemiologist Dr. David Sackett, formerly of McMaster University in Canada and now of Oxford University in England and co-editor of the new journal *Evidence-Based Medicine*, concluded in the 1960s that there were perhaps two physicians in Canada capable of conducting a proper randomized controlled trial.[21] Things have not changed greatly since.

One reason is that the practice of health care is an art as well as a science and much remains unknown. We now look at the art and science and philosophy of the chiropractic profession, and start with a brief history.

References

1 Cherkin DC, Mootz RD, eds. Chiropractic in the United States: training, practice and research. Rockville, Maryland: Agency for Health Care Policy and Research, Public Health Service, U.S. Department of Health and Human Services, 1997; AHCPR Publication No. 98–N002.

2 Gordon NP, Sobel DS, et al. Use of and interest in alternative therapies among adult primary care clinicians and adult members in a large health maintenance organization. West J Med 1998;169:153–61

3 Bigos S, Bowyer O, Braen G, et al. Acute low-back problems in adults. Clinical practice guideline No.14. Rockville, MD: Agency for Health Care Policy and Research, Public Health Service, U.S. Department of Health and Human Services, 1994; AHCPR Publication No. 95–0642.

4 Rosen M, Breen A, et al. Management guidelines for back pain. Appendix B in Report of a clinical standards advisory group committee on back pain. London, England: Her Majesty's Stationery Office (HMSO), 1994.

5 AMA pocket guide to back pain. New York: Random House, 1995.

6 Jarvis W. Foreword. In: Magner G. Chiropractic: the victim's perspective. Amhurst, New York: Prometheus Books, 1994: viii.

7 Cassidy JD, Bowen V. Macroscopic and microscopic anatomy of the sacroiliac joint from embryonic life Until the eighth decade. Spine 1981;6:620–8.

8 Cassidy JD, Mierau DR, et al. Sacroiliac Joint Dysfunction and Low-back Pain in School Aged Children. J Manip Physiol Ther 1984;7:81–4.

9 Giles LGF. Lumbo-sacral and cervical zygapophyseal joint inclusions. Man Med 1986;2:89–92, and other references there noted.

10 Cramer GD, Howe J, et al. Morphometric comparison of computed tomography to magnetic resonance imaging in the evaluation of the lumbar intervertebral foramin. Clin Anatomy 1984;7:173–80.

11 Mitchell BS, Humphreys BK, Sullivan E. Attachments of the ligamentum nuchae to cervical posterior spinal Dura and the lateral part of the occipital bone. J Manip Physiol Ther 1998;21:145–8.

12 Nilsson N. The Prevalence of Cervicogenic Headache in a Random Population Sample of 20-59 Year Olds. Spine 1995;20:1884–8.

13 Nilsson N, Christensen HW, et al. The effect of spinal manipulation in the treatment of cervicogenic headache. J Manip Physiol Ther 1997;20:326–30.

14 Waddell G, Feder G, et al. Low-back pain evidence review. London, England: Royal College of General Practitioners, 1996.

15 Katz M. Absurd claims by chiropractors clear new path for orthopractic. Med Post 1994 May.

16 Katz M. Presentation to Ontario Medical Association. Toronto, Ontario: May 27, 1994; taped transcript.

17 Hasselberg PD. Chiropractic in New Zealand: report of the Commission of Inquiry. Wellington, New Zealand: Government Printer, 1979:Chapter 23.

18 Smith R. Where is the wisdom . . . ? The poverty of medical evidence. Br Med J 1991;303:798–9.

19 Kirkaldy-Willis WH, Cassidy JD. Spinal manipulation in the treatment of low-back pain. Can Fam Phys 1985;31:535–40.

20 Haldeman S, Chapman-Smith D, Petersen DM, eds. Guidelines for chiropractic quality assurance and practice parameters: Proceedings of the Mercy Center Consensus Conference. Gaithersburg, Maryland: Aspen Publishers, 1993:Chapter 13.

21 Rachlis MD, Kushner C. Second opinion: what's wrong with Canada's health care system and how to fix it. Toronto, Ontario, Canada: Collins, 1989: 251.

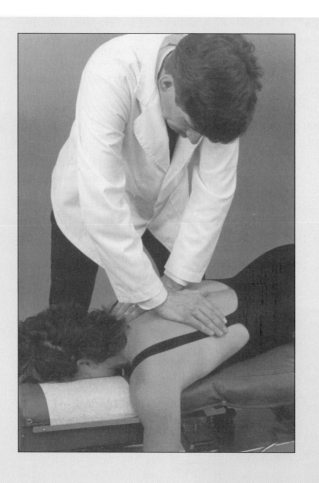

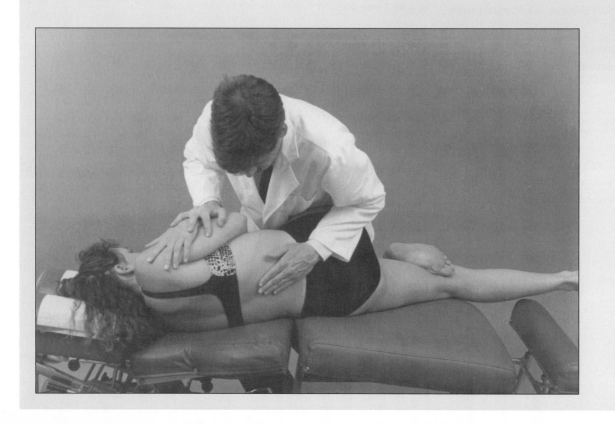

CHAPTER 2

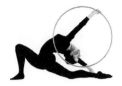

CHIROPRACTIC HISTORY

A. Introduction

In recent years spinal manipulation and the chiropractic profession "have gained a legitimacy in the United States health care system that until very recently seemed unimaginable," say Cherkin and Mootz in their foreword to the 1997 U.S. government-commissioned report on chiropractic titled *Chiropractic in the United States: Training, Practice and Research*[1] already referred to in Chapter 1.

This new level of acceptance is an international development. At the University of Odense in Denmark, chiropractic and medical students take the same basic science courses for three years before entering separate streams for clinical training. In countries where chiropractic educational programs began in the 1990s, such as Brazil, Italy and Korea, many chiropractic students are medical doctors.

Why has there been such a history of conflict between medicine and chiropractic? How and why has that changed? These are questions of interest not only to chiropractors and chiropractic students, but also patients, medical doctors and other health professionals. This chapter addresses these questions in the context of a brief history of the chiropractic profession. For a more complete history see *Chiropractic: History and Evolution of a New Profession* by Professor Walter Wardwell,[2] a sociologist who has studied the chiropractic profession since his Harvard doctoral thesis on the profession in 1951; and other fine histories by Moore,[3] a history professor from Radford University, Virginia, and Keating,[4] a psychologist and historian on faculty at the Los Angeles College of Chiropractic.

B. Beginnings

The chiropractic profession was founded in Davenport, Iowa, in 1895 by Daniel David Palmer, who had practiced magnetic healing in the years prior to this. His new focus was spinal adjustment or manipulation. An early patient, the Rev. Samuel Weed, suggested the name of the profession, which is derived from the Greek words *praxis* and *cheir* meaning practice by hand.

Palmer had no formal training but subscribed to the medical journals of the day. Those who have studied his writings conclude that he was unusually well-informed on major developments in anatomy and physiology in Europe and North America, indeed that "very few medical practitioners at his time in America could claim to be so well read."[5] He founded the Palmer School of Chiropractic in Davenport in 1897 and this remains one of the major chiropractic colleges today.

The Carver-Denny School of Chiropractic in Oklahoma City, circa 1910.

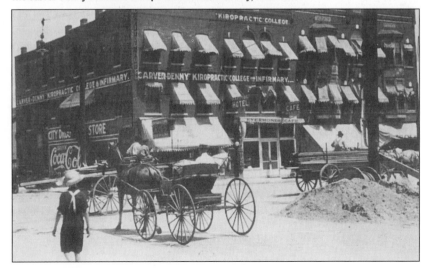

At this time, the beginning of the twentieth century, all health care was an art or craft more than an organized body of knowledge. There was little integration of science into education and treatment methods. The medical profession had not developed the dominant and respected role in health care it now enjoys. (This only happened in the U.S. after the 1910 Flexner Report condemned most medical education and led to major new funding and reforms.)

Chiropractic was only one of many new groups of healers that emerged at that time—bonesetters, herbal healers, homeopaths, hydro-healers, magnetic healers, osteopaths, Thompsonians, etc. It has proved to be one of the strongest survivors and is now taught and practiced throughout the world.

C. The Era of Conflict with Medicine

A third of the members of Palmer's first graduating class were medical doctors and G.H. Patchin, another physician, helped Palmer edit his primary text, *The Chiropractor's Adjuster.*[6]

But there were plain reasons for conflict between this new profession and medicine. Over the next 75 years these remained and included:

1. **Educational Standards**. During the period 1910 to 1950 U.S. medicine greatly improved and consolidated its standards and position in society, buttressed by major funding from the government and private foundations. Chiropractic education remained immature—in terms of entrance standards, program quality and length (the Palmer School only converted from an 18 months course to a 4 year program in 1949), faculty, accreditation and funding. Education remained a tuition-driven private enterprise.

2. **Spirit of Competitiveness**. Frankly speaking, both medicine and chiropractic set themselves up for a fight—and history suggests it benefited them both. Chiropractors claimed to have an alternative and superior fundamental approach to health. Medical doctors, they charged, merely treated symp-

---

Chiropractic History— Key Dates

1895 • D.D. Palmer commences practice as a "chiropractor" in Davenport, Iowa.

1897 • The Palmer School of Chiropractic, the first chiropractic educational institution, opens.

1905 • Minnesota becomes the first U.S. state to recognize and license the practice of chiropractic. Louisiana became the last state in 1974.

1923 • Alberta becomes the first province to license chiropractic practice in Canada. Ontario follows in 1925. Newfoundland is the last province, in 1992.

1933 • The U.S. Council of State Chiropractic Examining Boards is established with a mandate to provide unified standards for licensure. Renamed the Federation of Chiropractic Licensing Boards (FCLB) in 1974.

1939 • The Canton of Zurich, Switzerland, becomes the first jurisdiction outside North America to license the practice of chiropractic.

1944 • The Foundation for Chiropractic Education and Research (FCER) is established and, to the present time, is the profession's foremost agency for funding of postgraduate scholarship and research.

1963 • The U.S. National Board of Chiropractic Examiners (NBCE) is established to promote consistency and reciprocity between state examining boards.

1974 • The U.S. Council on Chiropractic Education (CCE) is recognized by the federal government as the accrediting agency for schools of chiropractic. This leads to the development of affiliated accrediting

agencies in Canada, Europe and Australia/New Zealand.

1979 • *Chiropractic in New Zealand*, the report of the NZ Commission of Inquiry into Chiropractic, is published. This was the first government commission to adopt a full judicial procedure, hearing evidence on oath and subject to cross-examination when examining patients, chiropractors, medical doctors and others on the role of the chiropractic profession. The Commission's recommendations strongly endorse chiropractic services and call for medical cooperation. The report has a major impact internationally.

1987 • Final judgment in the *Wilk vs American Medical Association* case entered, opening the way for much greater cooperation between medical and chiropractic doctors in education, research and practice in the U.S. and, as a result, internationally.

1988 • World Federation of Chiropractic (WFC) is formed. The WFC, whose members are national associations of chiropractors in over 70 countries, is admitted into official relations with the World Health Organization (WHO) as a non-governmental organization or NGO in January 1997.

1993 • The *Manga Report* in Canada, the first government-commissioned report by health economists looking at the cost-effectiveness of chiropractic services, recommends a primary role for chiropractors with back pain patients on grounds of safety, cost-effectiveness and patient preference, and concludes toms with the remedy of the day. Chiropractors understood the real cause of most ill health—malpositioned spinal vertebrae interfering with the nervous system and thereby obstructing the body's own natural or innate healing power. Patients should abandon drugs, surgery, and medical doctors and get all of their primary health care from chiropractors.

Medical doctors, in their turn, needed targets to build their credibility, unity, and the economic and political control of health care in the early twentieth century. Smith-Cunnien has shown that medical criticism of chiropractic has not been consistent, which is what one would have expected if medical criticism was really about chiropractic itself. Criticism was strongest when medicine needed new unity or came under attack—for example when the American Medical Association was first building real unity and strength from 1908 to 1924, and then when proposals were made for third

party funding of medical care in 1961 to 1976, proposals that would diminish medical control of the relationship with the patient.[7] Chiropractic, because of its combative nature and undeveloped status, was the perfect target.

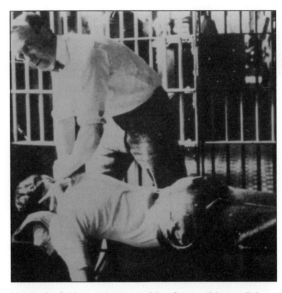

Hundreds of chiropractors served time for practicing medicine without a licence in the early years. Many of these continued treating inmates, jailors and the public. Here, Dr Fred Kotney adjusts a patient in his jail cell in Los Angeles, circa 1921.

this will save hundreds of millions annually in direct health care costs and work disability payments.

1994 • Government-sponsored expert panels developing evidence-based guidelines for the management of patients with back pain in the U.S. (Agency for Health Care Policy and Research[1]) and the U.K. (Clinical Standards Advisory Group[2]) provide the first authoritative reports that manipulation is a proven and preferred treatment approach for most acute low-back pain patients.

1996 • U.S. government begins official funding support for an ongoing agenda for chiropractic research. To continue this agenda the Consortial Center for Chiropractic Research is formed in 1997, comprising chiropractic schools, university research departments and federal government agencies, and is based at Palmer College of Chiropractic.

References

1 Bigos S, Bowyer O, Braen G, et al. Acute low-back problems in adults. Clinical practice guideline No.14. Rockville, Maryland: Agency for Health Care Policy and Research, Public Health Service, U.S. Department of Health and Human Services, 1994, AHCPR Publication No. 95-0642.

2 Rosen M, Breen A, et al. Management guidelines for back pain. Appendix B in Report of a clinical standards advisory group committee on back pain. London, England: Her Majesty's Stationery Office (HMSO), 1994.

Use of an early chiropractic table and technique demonstrated circa 1906 by Bartlett Joshua (BJ) Palmer, son of the founder of the profession, Daniel David (DD) Palmer.

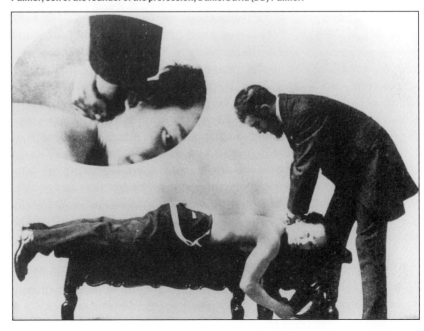

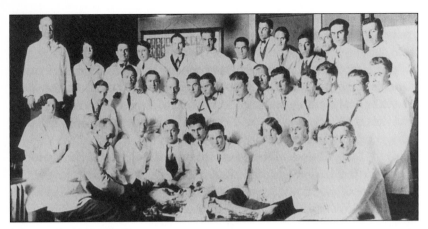

A class receives instruction in anatomy at Central States Chiropractic College, Indianapolis, Indiana, circa 1925.

3. **Excesses and Over-enthusiasm**. As the battle joined, each profession exposed itself through overclaim and overreaction. Chiropractors lionized their new profession, sometimes claiming spiritual authority. Palmer's son, Bartlett Joshua Palmer, was a courageous and vital leader for his profession in his generation, but given to such rhetoric and showmanship that he discredited the profession with medical authorities at the same time as he built it with chiropractors and the U.S. public. In the U.S. he split the profession into a vocal minority that would have no common ground with medicine and a growing mainstream that set about developing mature standards of education and practice. In Canada he set the profession back a generation by testifying to a Royal Commission in 1915 that "diagnosis was unnecessary, analysis of blood and urine samples was of no value," and that "bacteriology was the greatest of all gigantic farces ever invented for ignorance and incompetency."[8]

B.J. Palmer's counterparts for medicine were Morris Fishbein, Secretary of the American Medical Association (AMA) and editor of its journal from 1924 to 1949, and Doyle Taylor. Fishbein portrayed chiropractors as an "unscientific cult" and "rabid dogs" in what Wardwell calls "a campaign of vitriolic propaganda" against the profession.[9] He finally became too extreme even for the AMA which, as reported in *Harpers*[10] at the time, "withdrew its seal of acceptance . . . and kicked him into the street" because "physicians who were interested in something besides their fees resented their identification with his low-comedy routine."

Doyle Taylor, Director of the AMA Department of Investigation, was the driving force behind a McCarthy-like Committee on Quackery from 1963 which pursued the avowed and illegal goal of creating a health care monopoly for medicine that would eliminate the chiropractic profession. Many years later this became the subject of the landmark case of *Wilk and others vs. American Medical Association and others* in which a federal appeals court:

a) Found the AMA guilty of an illegal conspiracy "of systematic long-term wrongdoing and intent to destroy a licensed profession."

b) Found that this was based upon an extensive misinformation campaign portraying chiropractic as "unscientific" and "cultist" and being incompatible with modern medical practice. Tactics included suppressing research favorable to chiropractic, undermining chiropractic education, using new ethical rulings to prevent cooperation between medical doctors and chiropractors in education, practice and research and subverting a 1967 U.S. government inquiry into the merits of chiropractic.

The court gave judgment against the AMA, including a multi-million dollar award of costs and a permanent injunction or restraining order in these terms:

"The AMA, its officers, agents and employees, and all persons who act in active concert with any of them are hereby permanently enjoined from restricting, regulating or impeding . . . the freedom of any AMA member or any institution or hospital to make an individual decision as to whether or not that AMA member, institution, or hospital, shall professionally associate with chiropractors, chiropractic students, or chiropractic institutions."[11]

At the same time there were settlements with other defendants in the case, including the American Hospital Association, the American College of Surgeons, the American College of Radiology and the Joint Committee on Accreditation of Hospitals. The *Wilk Case*, filed in 1976, was of major significance in ushering in the present era of cooperation.

The court directed that the injunction be sent to all AMA members and published in the *Journal of the American Medical Association (JAMA)*, and there was immediately a significant increase in cooperation in practice, education and research. Medical specialists who had been reluctant to join editorial boards on chiropractic publications, refer patients to chiropractors or work in partnership with them, now did so.

4. **Economic/Legal/Political Issues**. Two generations of American chiropractors were prosecuted for practicing medicine without a license during the first half of the century, and many went to jail. The first state to license the practice of chiropractic was Minnesota in 1905, the last was Louisiana in 1974. The common picture in these battles was chiropractors and their patients opposed by the medical profession, but ultimately prevailing. These struggles kept the professions apart.

5. **Terminology.** This was divisive for two reasons. Firstly, chiropractors developed different terminology to defend themselves in court. They did not *diagnose* but rather performed a *spinal analysis,* and they did not offer *treatment* but *spinal corrections.* They were therefore practicing a separate profession, they argued, not medicine without a license.

Secondly, as with any profession, chiropractic adopted and preferred its own terms of art. A chiropractor gave a *spinal adjustment* rather than a *manipulation,* and the spinal problem treated was a *subluxation.* A major problem with the latter term was that the chiropractic definition (a joint dysfunction) contradicted the medical one (a significant joint displacement visible on x-ray). Medical doctors heard chiropractors saying they did not diagnose and did not treat conditions, but that they corrected subluxations —in circumstances when a medically-defined subluxation was not present. This provided fertile ground for dispute.

6. **Spinal Manipulation**. A further surprisingly strong reason for conflict was the form of treatment adopted by the chiropractic profession—whether called joint adjustment or manipulation. This has never been a part of medical education. In eighteenth and nineteenth century Europe manipulation was provided by lay bonesetters and always attracted medical hostility.

The medical profession has turned on its own few members who have practiced manipulation with as much criticism as it has given chiropractors. At the most thorough government inquiry into chiropractic anywhere, in New Zealand in 1978-79, the position of the New Zealand Medical Association (NZMA) was that no patient should receive spinal manipulation from anyone for anything. Manipulation was dangerous, ineffective and wrongheaded. NZMA member Dr. James Fisk, who had written one of the definitive medical texts on manipulation, was disowned and not called as a witness. Dr. James Cyriax in the U.K., Dr. John Mennell in the U.S., and Dr. John Bourdillon in Canada all encountered similar resistance throughout their careers into the 1980s.

This has all changed with medicine recognizing manipulation as a first line of treatment for most patients with back pain; but that change is recent. If one weighs all of the reasons for the era of conflict between medicine and chiropractic, the fact that chiropractors used manipulation—a treatment approach most medical doctors knew nothing about and that was apparently aimed at mechanical joint problems that could not be objectively seen or measured by medical diagnostic methods—was as significant as any other.

D. The 1970s—the Winds of Change

Until the end of the 1970s the chiropractic profession was still establishing its full infrastructure:

1. The legal right to practice and establish licensing legislation in all U.S. states and then internationally.

2. Sound educational standards and government-recognized accrediting agencies that guaranteed these standards.

3. A credible research agenda, with appropriately qualified research scientists and peer-reviewed scientific journals.

It took this long because the profession worked in isolation from medicine and the mainstream health care system. It enjoyed no public funding. (Pause to reflect upon the profound effect there would be on medical education and research if there was no public fund-

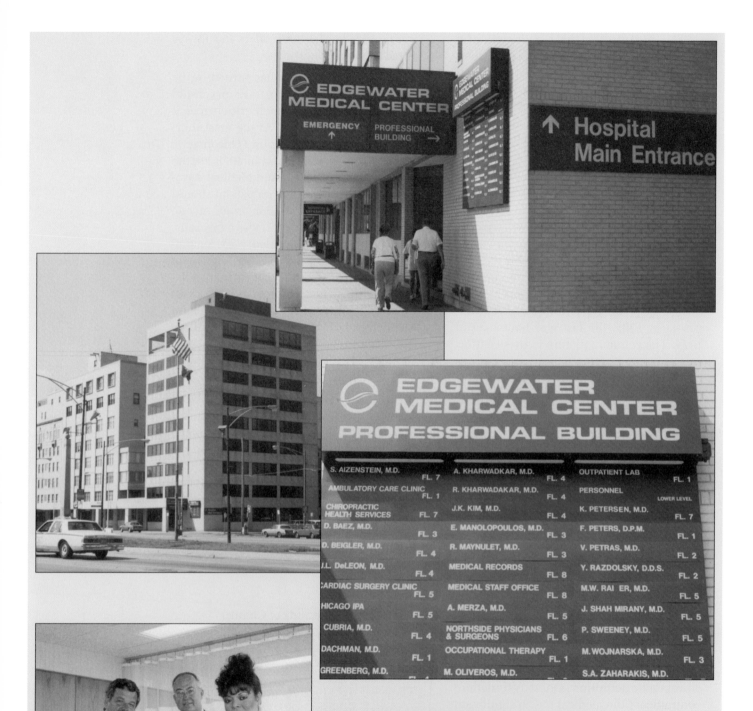

EDGEWATER MEDICAL CENTER PROFESSIONAL BUILDING		
S. AIZENSTEIN, M.D. FL. 7	A. KHARWADKAR, M.D. FL. 4	OUTPATIENT LAB FL. 1
AMBULATORY CARE CLINIC FL. 1	R. KHARWADAKAR, M.D. FL. 4	PERSONNEL LOWER LEVEL
CHIROPRACTIC HEALTH SERVICES FL. 7	J.K. KIM, M.D. FL. 4	K. PETERSEN, M.D. FL. 7
D. BAEZ, M.D. FL. 3	E. MANOLOPOULOS, M.D. FL. 3	F. PETERS, D.P.M. FL. 1
D. BEIGLER, M.D. FL. 4	R. MAYNULET, M.D. FL. 3	V. PETRAS, M.D. FL. 2
J.L. DeLEON, M.D. FL. 4	MEDICAL RECORDS FL. 8	Y. RAZDOLSKY, D.D.S. FL. 2
CARDIAC SURGERY CLINIC FL. 5	MEDICAL STAFF OFFICE FL. 8	M.W. RAI ER, M.D. FL. 5
CHICAGO IPA FL. 5	A. MERZA, M.D. FL. 5	J. SHAH MIRANY, M.D. FL. 5
CUBRIA, M.D. FL. 4	NORTHSIDE PHYSICIANS & SURGEONS FL. 6	P. SWEENEY, M.D. FL. 5
DACHMAN, M.D. FL. 1	OCCUPATIONAL THERAPY FL. 1	M. WOJNARSKA, M.D. FL. 3
GREENBERG, M.D.	M. OLIVEROS, M.D.	S.A. ZAHARAKIS, M.D.

Since 1991 the Edgewater Medical Center, a Chicago hospital, has had a Chiropractic Health Services Department, and upon admission many patients receive collaborative chiropractic and medical evaluation and care. Chiropractic students from the National College of Chiropractic have received part of their clinical training at EMC since 1995.

Pictured, *left,* are patient Dorothea Nelson (seated), and three staff members who co-manage her care. From left: Anton Riffling, DC, chiropractor, Andrew Cubria, MD, cardiologist, and Betty Graham, DC, chiropractor.

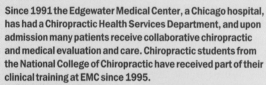

ing.) Because the practice of chiropractic made little use of technology and no use of drugs, the profession had no strong financial allies. (Pause to consider medicine with no support from the pharmaceutical industry.) Chiropractic was both isolated and opposed. It is true to add that the profession aggravated its situation with internal rivalries and conflict.

By the late 1970s many signs of maturity and imminent change were evident:

1. In 1974 the U.S. government formally recognized the Council on Chiropractic Education (CCE) as the accrediting agency for chiropractic educational institutions.

2. In 1975 chiropractic researchers were invited to the first U.S. federally-funded research conference on chiropractic and spinal manipulation, held at the National Institutes of Health, Bethesda, Maryland.[12]

3. In 1979 the first major interdisciplinary text with chiropractic and medical authors was released, *Modern Developments in the Principles and Practice of Chiropractic,*[13] edited by Scott Haldeman, DC, MD, PhD, a chiropractor and neurologist.

4. In the same year the *Journal of Manipulative and Physiological Therapeutics (JMPT)*, the first peer-reviewed chiropractic journal, began publication.

5. In 1977 in Australia,[14] and 1979 in New Zealand,[15] the first comprehensive government commissions of inquiry into chiropractic delivered independent findings strongly supportive of the contemporary chiropractic profession, and calling for close cooperation between chiropractic and medicine in education and practice in the public interest.

Government inquiries, like research, are of widely varying quality and some deserve little credibility. Of importance are the qualifications of the commissioners, the terms of reference, the procedures adopted for hearing and testing evidence and the degree of opportunity to hear all relevant evidence.

On these criteria the most comprehensive and detailed independent examination of chiropractic ever undertaken was that in New Zealand in 1978/79. The Commission's report, *Chiropractic in New Zealand* (377 pages)[15] has obvious authority and balance.

It followed extensive investigations by the Commission conducted in New Zealand, the United States, Canada, England and Australia. For these reasons further details on the Commission, including its principal findings, are given in Table 1 on page 18. As you read these findings—independent assessments of the quality and maturity of chiropractic education and practice—remember that they were made 20 years ago.

In terms of the maturity and more widespread acceptance of the chiropractic profession, the winds of change were blowing firmly as the 1980s began.

E. The 1980s—New Common Ground with Medicine

Although all health professions have their trade associations and political and economic interests, most individual health professionals spend their daily lives in close personal contact with patients. Fundamentally they support the best interests of their patients. This is true of most medical doctors and chiropractors.

By the early 1980s the public had spoken clearly, providing this foundation for new common ground between the two professions:

1. There was wide public acceptance and use of chiropractic services, particularly for two of the three most common reasons the public uses health care services—headache and back pain.

2. As a large U.S. national survey from Stanford University has now confirmed, chiropractic patients generally use both chiropractic and medical services and want cooperation between their chosen health care providers.[16]

3. The medical profession acknowledged that their approach to management of back pain was—as patients had demonstrated with their choices—largely ineffective. Rest, and medication and a focus on the herniated disc and other structural pathology were inappropriate. Back pain was usually a 'biopsychosocial' problem. (For the meaning of this see page 109.) Most patients needed early return to normal activities, reassurance, non-prescription drugs and/or manipulation for pain relief and correction of functional pathology in joints and muscles. This was consistent with a chiropractic approach.

continued on page 21

Table 1 **The New Zealand Commission of Inquiry—1977/78. One of several government commissions to investigate the chiropractic profession, the New Zealand Commission of Inquiry is regarded as having delivered the most detailed and exhaustive report.**

Terms of Reference:

To consider whether government health and accident compensation benefits should be made available for chiropractic services having regard to the practice and philosophy of chiropractic, its scientific and educational basis, whether it constituted a separate and distinct healing art, and the contribution it could make to New Zealand health services.

Membership:
Brian D. Inglis, Q.C., B.A. J.D. LL.D. Chairman. A senior litigation lawyer, and Professor of Law, Victoria University, Wellington. Now a judge.
Betty Fraser, M.B.E., M.A. a prominent educationalist.
Bruce R. Penfold, M.Sc., Ph.D., F.R.S.N.Z. Professor of Chemistry, University of Canterbury.

Procedure:

Public judicial hearings. Evidence given orally, but on basis of a written submission filed with the Commission and available to principal parties at least 30 days prior to allow time for informed cross-examination. On oath and subject to examination by all interested parties, including legal counsel representing the chiropractic, medical and physiotherapy professions.

Evidence was recorded verbatim and appears in a 3638 page typewritten transcript. This record assisted cross examination and proper evaluation of evidence, and is referenced by the Commission in its report in support of findings made.

In addition there were some private hearings, impromptu visits to chiropractic practices to observe the profession at work, and personal investigation of chiropractic, medicine, and physiotherapy in the United States, Canada, England and Australia—see Report for details.

Depth of Inquiry:

The Commission's opportunity to hear evidence was extremely wide, since there were no restraints on time, and both medicine and chiropractic worldwide saw this as the test case for chiropractic. Consumer, chiropractic, medical and physiotherapy witnesses from the United States, Europe, Canada and Australia came to give evidence at the New Zealand hearings. The Commission and all parties contemplated an inquiry of under 6 months. The inquiry in fact required over 18 months.

Principal Findings: *(For complete findings see report, Chapter 1)*

The following principal findings appear in the introduction to the Report:

• Modern chiropractic is far from being an "unscientific cult."

• Chiropractic is a branch of the healing arts specializing in the correction by spinal manual therapy of what chiropractors identify as biomechanical disorders of the spinal column. They carry out spinal diagnosis and therapy at a sophisticated and refined level.

• Chiropractors are the only health practitioners who are necessarily equipped by their education and training to carry out spinal manual therapy.

• General medical practitioners and physiotherapists have no adequate training in spinal manual therapy, though a few have acquired skill in it subsequent to graduation.

• Spinal manual therapy in the hands of a registered chiropractor is safe.

• The education and training of a registered chiropractor are sufficient to enable him to determine whether there are contra-indications to spinal manual therapy in a particular case, and whether the patient should have medical care instead of or as well as chiropractic care.

• Spinal manual therapy can be effective in relieving musculo-skeletal symptoms such as back pain, and other symptoms known to respond to such therapy, such as migraine.

• In a limited number of cases where there are organic and/or visceral symptoms, chiropractic treatment may provide relief, but this is unpredictable, and in such cases the patient should be under concurrent medical care if that is practicable.

• Although the precise nature of the biomechanical dysfunction which chiropractors claim to treat has not yet been demonstrated scientifically, and although the precise reasons why spinal manual therapy provides relief have not yet been scientifically explained, chiropractors have reasonable grounds based on clinical evidence for their belief that symptoms of the kind described above can respond beneficially to spinal manual therapy.

• Chiropractors do not provide an alternative comprehensive system of health care, and should not hold themselves out as doing so.

• In the public interest and in the interests of patients there must be no impediment to full professional cooperation between chiropractors and medical practitioners.

• It is wrong that the present law, or any medical ethical rules, should have the effect that a patient can receive spinal manual therapy which is subsidised by a health benefit only from those health professionals least well qualified to deliver it.

• The responsibility for spinal manual therapy training, because of its specialised nature, should lie with the chiropractic profession. Part-time or vacation courses in spinal manual therapy for other health professionals should not be encouraged.

The Commission, in answer to the basic question before it, recommended government funding for chiropractic services. There were also recommendations concerning discipline, interprofessional ethics, hospital access and government funded research to be conducted jointly by the chiropractic and medical professions. This Report remains the best reading for impartial conclusions on all aspects of the chiropractic profession.

CHIROPRACTIC
IN NEW ZEALAND

REPORT OF THE
COMMISSION OF INQUIRY

1979

*Presented to the House of Representatives by Command of
His Excellency the Governor-General*

BY AUTHORITY:
F. D. HASSELBERG, GOVERNMENT PRINTER, WELLINGTON, NEW ZEALAND—1979
Price $7.65

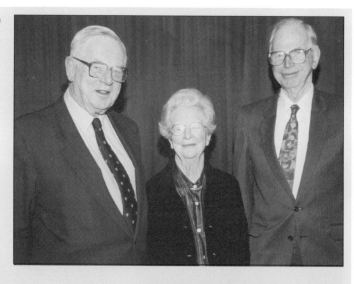

right: **Pictured from left are NZ Commissioners Judge B. Donald Inglis, Chairman, Betty Fraser and Professor Bruce Penfold.**

left: **Richard Craddock, QC, lead counsel for the NZ Chiropractors' Association;** *right:* **witness Scott Haldeman, MD DC PhD, a Los Angeles neurologist and chiropractor;** *below:* **witness Robin McKenzie, PT, a New Zealand physiotherapist.**

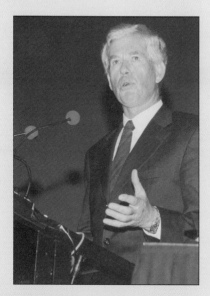

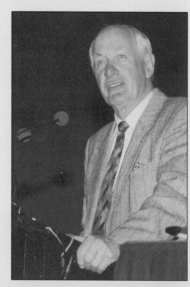

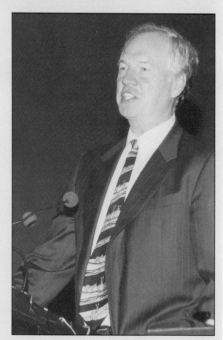

below: **Patients who gave evidence, seen here recounting their experiences, included** *left:* **Mrs. Inez Newton, who was completely disabled by back pain and sciatica for 12 months before opting for chiropractic care and making a full recovery, and** *right:* **Mr. Paddy Sheehy, seen here with his chiropractor Dr. Ronald Sim. Mr. Sheehy had received medical advice he would be confined to a wheelchair for life after a motor-vehicle accident because of neurological injuries, but subsequently recovered in full. Standing on the table (at center) is his subsequent award as senior champion at his local tennis club.**

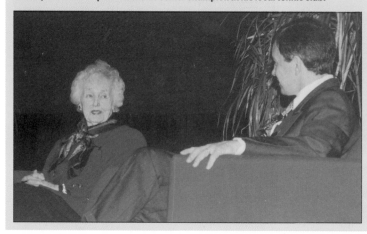

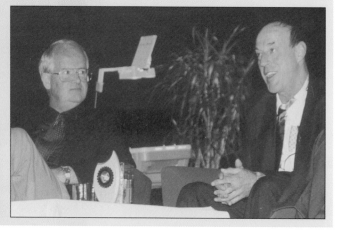

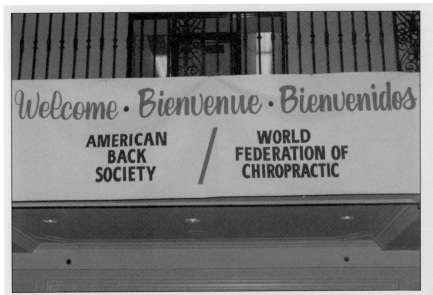

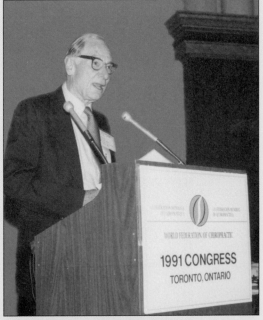

Professor William Kirkaldy-Willis, an orthopedic surgeon and President, American Back Society (ABS), addresses 750 chiropractic and medical doctors in 1991 in Toronto at a joint meeting of the ABS and the World Federation of Chiropractic, and calls for better cooperation between the medical and chiropractic professions in the interests of patients and improved care.

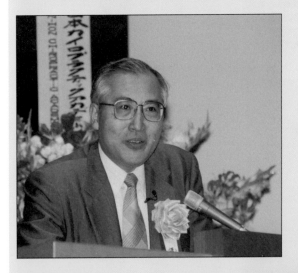

Akio Sato, MD, PhD, a Japanese neurophysiologist, addresses 1,800 members of an interdisciplinary audience at the World Federation of Chiropractic's 4th Biennial Congress in Tokyo in 1997.

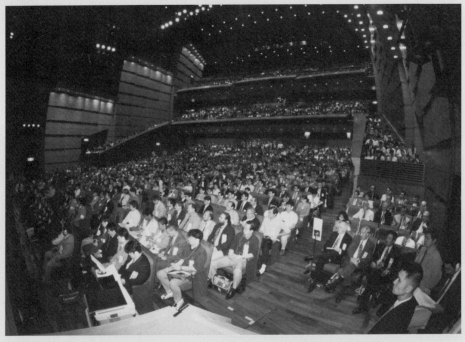

4. Chiropractors, likewise, had shed their earlier simplistic claim that all back pain was the result of spinal subluxation. When medical doctors had said back pain was either the result of structural pathology or, in the absence of that, was largely psychological, and chiropractors had said it was caused by subluxation, there was no basis for understanding. Now they shared the same model.

6. The mainstream chiropractic profession reacted to higher educational qualifications, the responsibilities of licensure, the wishes of patients, and the increasing inter-referral of patients and contact with the medical profession by moderating its claims as to the scope of practice of chiropractic. Chiropractic was not an alternative approach to healing based on theories inconsistent with modern medicine. It was different in emphasis only and complementary. It focused on manual and other non-invasive treatments primarily for neuromusculoskeletal disorders

The new spirit of cooperation, despite continuing controversy at the political level, was evident. In education the faculty of chiropractic colleges now included medical doctors and basic scientists, many of whom also held appointments at medical schools. At the postgraduate level, chiropractors were now admitted to the meetings of medical and interdisciplinary organizations such as the American Back Society in the U.S. and the Physical Medicine Research Foundation in Canada.

In research there was growing cooperation. In 1984, reflecting the history of conflict, the journal *Manual Medicine* had replied to Dr. Howard Vernon, a chiropractic researcher submitting a trial for publication, with the brief and remarkably frank response that the journal "does not publish any research from a chiropractic source." But by 1986, two years later, it did.

In 1985 the *Canadian Family Physician*, the official journal of the Royal College of Family Physicians of Canada, published *Spinal Manipulation in the Treatment of Low-Back Pain* by Kirkaldy-Willis and Cassidy, an orthopedic surgeon and a chiropractor who reported excellent results from their work together at the Royal University Hospital in Saskatoon and encouraged much greater cooperation between family physicians and doctors of chiropractic.[17] In the U.S. medical researchers at the RAND Corpora-

tion, and in the U.K. epidemiologists funded by the Medical Research Council, were working with chiropractic researchers on a consensus study[18] and a major clinical trial[19] that would support the appropriateness and effectiveness of manipulation for acute and chronic back pain. In Perth, Australia, Lynton Giles, DC, PhD, was producing anatomical research at the University of Western Australia that was being published in leading medical journals.[20,21]

In daily practice there was now steady referral of patients by medical doctors in all countries where the chiropractic profession was established. A 1989 survey from the University of Toronto reported that, by the end of the 1980s, a clear majority of family physicians in Ontario (62%) were referring patients to chiropractors, and that nearly 1 in 10 (9.5%) were patients themselves. All family physicians with a chiropractor in the same building or mall were making referrals.[22] It was not until the 1990s, however, that it became usual for chiropractic and medical doctors to practice in the same clinic or hospital, increasingly in formal partnerships.

F. The 1990s—Reasons for Cooperation

In the 1990s there was quite dramatic growth in public and medical acceptance of chiropractic services. Main reasons for the acceptance of chiropractors into mainstream health care may be summarized as follows:

1. *Improved standards of chiropractic education*. In many countries chiropractic education has now been incorporated into the publicly-funded university system—for example Australia, Brazil, Canada, Denmark, England, South Africa and Wales. In the U.S. chiropractic colleges remain largely private but have minimum standards of governance and education established by the Council on Chiropractic Education, the government-recognized accrediting agency for the chiropractic profession.

2. *Improved standards of regulation of chiropractic practice*.

3. *The final judgment, after years of appeals, of the Wilk Case in 1987*. In the U.S. this finally made it possible for medical doctors to cooperate with chiropractors in all aspects of education, research and practice without fear of loss of hospital and other privileges essential to their practices and income.

4. *Articles favorable to chiropractic in medical*

journals published by medical associations. Examples include the *Annals of Internal Medicine*, American College of Physicians,[23],[24] *British Medical Journal*, British Medical Association,[19] and the *Canadian Family Physician*, Royal College of Family Physicians of Canada).[17] These publications have signaled to physicians that it is now safe and appropriate to work with chiropractors.

5. *Other research and clinical guidelines for practice.* Today almost every issue of *Spine*, the most respected medical journal in its

The new integration of chiropractic into mainstream health care services offers benefits to all—physicians, chiropractors and their mutual patients.

field worldwide and one that has an international editorial board, has chiropractic research. Government-sponsored evidence-based guidelines for practice in many countries, but most prominently in the U.S.[25] and the U.K. [26] in 1994, have recommended spinal manipulation as a first line approach to the management of most patients with acute back pain.

6. *Patient demand.* A better informed public that is taking more control of its health care is placing new demands on all health care providers, and requiring cooperation between medical and complementary and alternative health practitioners.

7. *The evolution of health care.* The dental and medical monopolies of 25 years ago have been replaced by health care systems that

include, regulate and fund many independent specialized professionals with whom dentists and medical doctors must work. Dentists see their patients also attending independent dental hygienists, denturists and dental nurses—and chiropractors for jaw problems. Medical doctors must work with acupuncturists, massage therapists, midwives, naturopaths, nurse practitioners and specialists, optometrists, osteopaths, podiatrists, many others—and chiropractors.

G. Further Examples of Government and Medical Acceptance

This historical review now closes with further recent examples of acceptance.

1. In the United States, federal government funding for chiropractic services, which has existed for many years under Medicare and Medicaid, has since 1995 been extended to programs for the military and their families. In addition since 1996 the government has established and funded a Consortial Center for Chiropractic Research comprising representatives of chiropractic schools, university research departments and federal government agencies. It is based at Palmer College of Chiropractic and has an ongoing national agenda for chiropractic research.

2. In Canada there is federal and provincial government funding for chiropractic services. The recent decision by York University, Toronto, to establish a school of chiropractic in affiliation with the Canadian Memorial Chiropractic College follows the example of the University of Quebec, which

Opening ceremonies for chiropractic clinics, *left*, at the Wellesley Central Hospital, Toronto, in August 1996 and, *right*, at the University of Waterloo in August 1997 in Ontario, Canada. These clinics, which are also clinical research centers, are affiliated with the Canadian Memorial Chiropractic College.

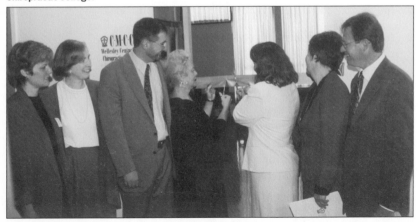
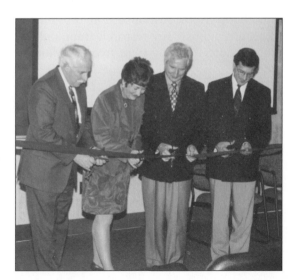

opened its school of chiropractic in Trois Rivières in 1993.

3. In the United Kingdom the British Medical Association (BMA) has actively supported the increased recognition and integration of chiropractic services into the British health care system that has occurred during the 1990s, on the grounds that many BMA members wish to refer patients to chiropractors.[27]

4. Internationally the World Health Organization's 1997 decision to admit the World Federation of Chiropractic (WFC), which represents national chiropractic associations from over 70 countries, into official relations as a non-governmental organization (NGO) is another sign of the evolution to acceptance. The WFC's application was supported by other health sector NGOs representing physicians (e.g. World Federation of Neurology), nurses (International Council of Nurses) and public health authorities (World Federation of Public Health Associations). Speaking on behalf of the World Health Organization (WHO) at a meeting in October 1998 at De La Salle University, Manila, the Philippines, Dr. N.V.K. Nair, Director, Health Infrastructure, WHO Regional Office for the Western Pacific explained to government and medical leaders:

"Chiropractic is an accepted form of healing to WHO. Its acceptance, recognition and availability is gradually spreading in the countries of the Western Pacific . . . I am aware of the hesitation in so-called modern medical circles to accept chiropractic as their partners in lessening the suffering from specific conditions, especially musculo-skeletal. Many forget the benefits of joining hands between modern and traditional medicine. . . . Times have changed and now it is the customer's demand which is the crucial factor."[28]

(*Traditional medicine*, rather than *complementary* or *alternative* medicine, is WHO's terminology for disciplines such as chiropractic and acupuncture. The practice of chiropractic was formally recognized by legislation in the Philippines in 1997 and De La Salle University now plans to open a school of chiropractic in conjunction with its schools of medicine and other health sciences.)

In some countries the evolution to acceptance is far from complete, principally because there are few or no chiropractors in practice. Indeed the practice of spinal manipulation remains a medical act in some European countries such as France, Hungary and Spain where there is still no legislation to recognize the chiropractic profession. But most of the root causes of conflict with medicine are gone and there is no medical specialty that can provide the public with the equivalent of chiropractic services. Chiropractic, like dentistry, is a diagnosing, primary contact profession that is complementary to medicine but with separate training and practice. The new integration of chiropractic into mainstream health care services offers benefits to all—medical doctors, chiropractors and their mutual patients.

References

1 Cherkin DC, Mootz RD, eds. Chiropractic in the United States: training, practice and research. National Technical Information Service, U.S. Department of Commerce, 1997; Document No. PB98111693.

2 Wardwell WL. Chiropractic: history and evolution of a new profession. St. Louis, Missouri: Mosby Year Book Inc, 1992.

3 Moore JS. Chiropractic in America: the history of a medical alternative. Baltimore, Maryland and London, England: Johns Hopkins University Press, 1993.

4 Keating JC. B.J. of Davenport: the early years of chiropractic. Davenport, Iowa: Association for the History of Chiropractic, 1997.

5 Gaucher-Peslherbe PL, Wiese G, Donahue J. Daniel David Palmer's medical library: the founder was into the literature. Chiro Hist 1995;15(2):63–9.

6 Palmer DD. The chiropractor's adjuster: The science, art and philosophy of chiropractic. Portland, Oregon: Portland Printing House, 1910. Available from the Palmer College of Chiropractic, Davenport, Iowa.

7 Smith-Cunnien SL. A profession of one's own. Lanham, New York: University Press of America, 1998.

8 Sutherland DC. Trial By Fire: Canadian Royal Commissions Investigate Chiropractic. Chiro Hist 1985;5:27–37.

9 Ref 2, supra, 161–2.

10 Mayer M. The rise and fall of Dr. Fishbein. Harpers 1949;199:76–85.

11 Wilk et al. v American Medical Association et al. U.S. Federal Court, Northern District of Illinois, Eastern Division No. 76C3777, Getzendanner J, Judgement dated August 27, 1987.

12 Goldstein M, ed. The research status of spinal manipulative therapy: a workshop on health at the National Institutes of Health. Bethesda, Maryland: U.S. Department of Health, Education and Welfare, 1975.

13 Haldeman S, ed. Modern developments in the principles and practice of chiropractic. New York: Appleton-Century-Crofts, 1979.

14 Report of the Committee of Inquiry into Chiropractic, Osteopathy, Homeopathy and Naturopathy (Webb Report). Canberra, Australia: Australian Government Publishing Service, 1977.

15 Hasselberg PD. Chiropractic in New Zealand. Report of the Commission of Inquiry into Chiropractic. Wellington, New Zealand: Government Printer, 1979.

16 Astin JA. Why patients use alternative medicine: results of a national study. JAMA 1998;279:1548–53.

17 Kirkaldy-Willis WH, Cassidy JD. Spinal Manipulation in the Treatment of Low-Back Pain. Can Fam Phys 1985;31:535–40.

18 Shekelle PG, Adams AH, et al. The Appropriateness of Spinal Manipulation for Low-Back Pain: Indications and Ratings by a Multidisciplinary Expert Panel. Santa Monica, California: RAND, 1991. Monograph No. R-4025/2–CCR/FCER.

19 Meade TW, Dyer S, et al. Low-back pain of mechanical origin: randomised comparison of chiropractic and hospital outpatient treatment. Br Med J 1990;300:1431–7.

20 Giles LGF, Taylor JR, Cockson A. Human zygapophysial joint synovial folds. Acta Anat 1986;126:110–4.

21 Giles LGF, Kaveri MJP. Immunohistochemical demonstration of nociceptors in the capsule and synovial folds of human zygapophysial joints. Br J Rheumatol 1987;26:362–4.

22 Patel-Christopher A. Family physicians and chiropractors: a need for better communication and cooperation (thesis). Toronto, Ontario: University of Toronto, 1990.

23 Shekelle G, Adams AH, et al. Spinal manipulation for low-back pain. Ann Intern Med 1992;117:590–8.

24 Shekelle PG, Coulter I, et al. Congruence between decisions: to initiate chiropractic spinal manipulation for low-back pain and appropriateness criteria in North America. Ann Intern Med 1998;129:9–17.

25 Bigos S, Bowyer O, Braen G, et al. Acute low-back problems in adults. Clinical Practice Guideline No.14. Rockville, Maryland: Agency for Health Care Policy and Research, Public Health Service, U.S. Department of Health and Human Services, 1994; AHCPR Publication No. 95-0642.

26 Rosen M, Breen A, et al. Management guidelines for back pain. Appendix B in Report of a clinical standards advisory group committee on back pain. London, England: Her Majesty's Stationery Office (HMSO), 1994.

27 Complementary medicine, new approaches to good practice. Oxford, England: British Medical Association, Oxford University Press, 1993.

28 Nair NVK. Introductory address at a symposium titled Chiropractic in Asia. Health Infrastructure, WHO Western Pacific Region. Manila, Philippines: De La Salle University, October 2, 1998.

CHAPTER 3

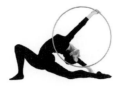

CURRENT STATUS OF THE PROFESSION

A. Introduction

The chiropractic profession was founded in 1895. The next 75 years saw consistent growth, first in the United States and Canada and then internationally. Throughout these years the chiropractic profession was still establishing its educational standards, its own scientific journals, texts, research organizations and legal right to practice. There was opposition from the medical profession. However in the last 25 years chiropractic has blossomed, becoming a large and mature profession that is established in over 60 countries throughout the world. This chapter reviews the current status of the profession in terms of size and professional organiza-

tion, law, education, literature, research funding for services, practice settings and postgraduate specialties

B. Professional Organization

1. **International Organizations**. In 1998 there were approximately 65,000 chiropractors practicing in the United States, approximately 90,000 internationally. It is estimated that by the year 2010 there will be 100,000 chiropractors in the United States, which would represent 1 for every 6 medical doctors, and 150,000 internationally. One significant development during the past 15 years has been the formation and growth of

• Countries with national chiropractic associations that are members of the World Federation of Chiropractic, a non-governmental organization (NGO) in official relations with the World Health Organization.

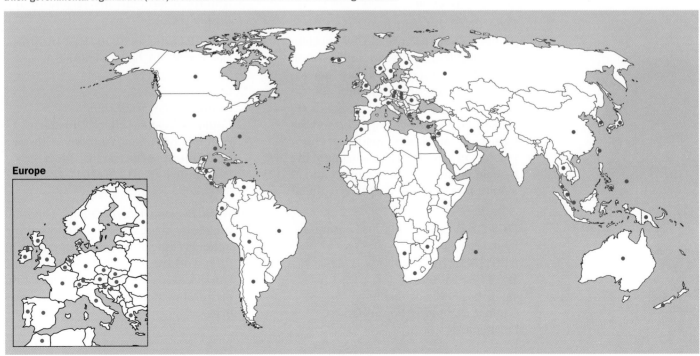

Europe

world organizations to coordinate the international development of chiropractic education, practice and research.

a) *World Federation of Chiropractic (WFC).* The WFC was founded in 1988, has secretariats in Toronto, Canada and Geneva, Switzerland, and its voting members are 70 national chiropractic associations from throughout the world. The WFC, which is in official relations with the World Health Organization (WHO) and is a member of the Council of International Organizations of Medical Sci-

FCER is the leading chiropractic research agency internationally and is funding research not only in North America but also in Asia, Europe and the Pacific.

ences (CIOMS), holds a biennial multidisciplinary congress presenting the leading original research from chiropractors worldwide. It is the profession's primary forum for developing a consistent basis for legal recognition, education and practice in all world regions.

WFC: 3080 Yonge Street, Suite 5065, Toronto Ontario M4N 3N1, Canada, tel: 416-484-9978, fax: 416-484-9665, email: worldfed@sympatico.ca, website: www.wfc.org. *Contact:* Mr. David Chapman-Smith, Secretary-General.

b) *Fédération International de Chiropratique Sportive (FICS).* FICS was established in 1986 and serves a similar role to the WFC in the specialized and increasingly important arena of sports chiropractic. It has coordinated postgraduate education in sports chiropractic and the greatly increased participation of chiropractors in sports medicine teams at the Barcelona and Atlanta Olympics and at many other national and international sporting competitions.

FICS: Ch. De la Joliette, 1006 Lausanne, Switzerland, tel: 011-41-21-612933, fax: 41-21-617-3016, email: fics@worldcom.ch. *Contact:* Daniele Bertamini, DC, President.

c) *Council on Chiropractic Education (CCE).* CCE, by itself, is not an international organization. It is the accrediting agency for chiropractic educational programs in the United States recognized by the U.S. government since 1974. However it structure and standards have been followed by similar CCEs in Australia, Canada and Europe and this has provided the basis for common educational standards internationally which are monitored by the various CCEs and the World Federation of Chiropractic.

CCE: 8049 N. 85th Way, Scottsdale, Arizona 85258-4321, USA, tel: 480-443-8877, fax: 480-483-7333, email: cce@adata.com. *Contact:* Paul Walker, PhD, Executive Director.

d) *Foundation for Chiropractic Education and Research (FCER).* FCER is also U.S.-based but is the leading chiropractic research agency internationally and has developed an international funding and project base. In many countries chiropractors are completing basic science doctoral degrees with the assistance of FCER fellowships and FCER is funding research not only in North America but also in Asia, Europe and the Pacific. Much of the private funding for research from individual chiropractors and chiropractic organizations is channeled through FCER.

FCER: P.O. Box 4689, 704 East 4th Street, Des Moines, IA, 50306-4689 USA, tel: 515-282-7118, fax: 515-282-3347, email: fcernow@aol.com. *Contacts:* Deanna L. Beck, Director of Administration, and Anthony L. Rosner, PhD, Director of Research. (Direct Boston line: 888-690-1378 or 617-734-3397.)

e) *World Regional Organizations.* There are professional organizations representing national associations of chiropractors in three world regions. These organizations work closely with the World Federation of Chiropractic but are not formally parts of it.

Asia—*Asian Chiropractic Federation (ACF)*. Room 1406 Jollibee Centre Building, Room 1406, San Miguel Avenue, Pasig City, Metro Manila, Philippines, tel: 011-63-2-633-4204, fax: 011-63-2-813-3059, email: jtuydc@evoserve.com. *Contact:* Jameson Uy, DC, President.

Europe—*European Chiropractors' Union (ECU)*. 9 Cross Deep Gardens, Twickenham, Middlesex, TW1 4QZ, England, tel: 011-441-81-891-2546, fax: 011-441-81-744-2902, email: ECUAnne@aol.com. *Contact: Anne Kemp, Executive Secretary.*

Latin America—*Federaçion Latino-Americano de Quiropractica (FLAQ)*. Gutenberg 133, Col. Anzures, C.P. 11590, Mexico DF, tel: 011-52-5-250-0433, fax: 011-52-5-203-5140. *Contact:* Enrique Benet-Canut, DC, President.

2. **North America**

   a) **National Associations**. The two largest national associations in the world are the American Chiropractic Association (ACA) and the Canadian Chiropractic Association (CCA). In the U.S. there is a second national association named the International Chiropractors' Association (ICA). The ACA and ICA conduct an increasing number of joint educational, public education and political action initiatives.

   As health care laws and rights and funding arrangements are mainly matters of state/provincial law in the U.S. and Canada rather than national law, chiropractors' first professional memberships are often with their state or provincial associations. U.S. state associations are separate in structure from the national associations and the federal organization is the Congress of Chiropractic State Associations (COCSA). In Canada the various provincial associations are divisions of the Canadian Chiropractic Association and therefore have no separate federal organization.

ACA: 1701 Clarendon Boulevard, Arlington, Virginia 22209, USA, tel: 703-276-8800, fax: 703-243-2593, email: memberinfo@americhiro.org, website: www.amerchiro.org. *Contact:* Mr. Garrett Cuneo, Executive Vice-President.

CCA: 1396 Eglinton Avenue West, Toronto, Ontario M6C 2E4, Canada, tel: 416-781-5656, fax: 416-781-7344, email: ccachiro@inforamp.net, website: www.inforamp.net/~ccachiro. *Contact:* Mr. Edward Barisa, Executive Director.

ICA: 1110 Glebe Road, Suite 1000, Arlington, Virginia 22201, USA, tel: 703-528-5000, fax: 703-528-5023, email: chiro@erols.com, website: www.chiropractic.org. *Contact:* Mr. Ronald Hendrickson, Executive Vice-President.

COCSA: P.O. Box 2054, Lexington, South Carolina 29071-2054 USA, tel: 803-356-6809, fax: 803-356-6226, email: jjordan@chirolink.com. *Contact:* Ms. Janet Jordan, Executive Director.

   b) **Educational Organizations**

      i) *Council on Chiropractic Education (CCE)*.
         8049 N. 85th Way, Scottsdale, Arizona 85258-4321, USA, tel: 602-443-8877, fax: 602-483-7333, email: cce@adata.com. *Contact*: Paul Walker, PhD, Executive Director).

      This is the U.S. national accrediting agency. For more information on the roles of this and CCE Canada see Chapter 4 titled "Education and Licensure".

ii) *Council on Chiropractic Education
(CCE Canada).*
6091 Gilbert Road, Suite 440,
Richmond, British Columbia
V7C 5L9, Canada,
tel: 1-604-278-3505,
fax: 1-604-940-9426,
email: Dnixdorf@netcom.ca.
Contact: Alex Guy, DC, President.

iii) *Association of Chiropractic Colleges
(ACC).*
4424 Montgomery Avenue, Suite
102, Bethesda, Maryland 20814,
USA,
tel: 301-652-5066,
fax: 301-913-9146,
email: obryonco@aol.com.
Contact: Mr. David O'Bryon,
Executive Director.

c) **Licensing Organizations**

i) *Federation of Chiropractic Licensing
Boards (FCLB).*
901 54th Avenue, Suite 101, Greely,
Colorado 80634, USA,
tel: 970-356-3500,
fax: 970-356-3599,
email: fclb@fclb.org,
website: www.fclb.org.
Contact: Donna Liewer, Executive
Director.

This is the federation of state licensing boards. It has an annual publication that summarizes useful information on the licensing of chiropractic
practice in each state—including
scope of practice, size and constitu-
tion of the regulatory board (e.g. how
many chiropractic, lay and medical
members), address of board, examination requirements, etc.

ii) *National Board of Chiropractic
Examiners (NBCE).*
901 54th Avenue, Greely, Colorado
80634, USA,
tel: 970-356-9100,
fax: 970-356-6134,
email: nbce@nbce.org,
website: www.NBCE.org/nbce.
Contact: Mr. Horace G. Elliott,
Executive Director.

The NBCE develops and administers
state and national board licensing
examinations. For more on this see
Chapter 4.

iii) *Canadian Federation of Chiropractic
Regulatory Boards (CFCRB).*
3080 Yonge Street, Toronto, Ontario
M4N 3N1, Canada,
tel: 416-486-0005,
fax: 416-486-1587,
email: pwaite@vcomsolutions.com,
Contact: Mr. Peter Waite, Executive
Director.

CRCFB has the same role in Canada as
the FCLB in the U.S.

iv) *Canadian Chiropractic Examining
Board (CCEB).*
1020 Centre Street North, Calgary,
Alberta T2E 2P9, Canada,
tel: 403-230-5997,
fax: 403-230-3321,
email: Dmcewen@cceb.ca.
Contact: Murray C. McEwen, DC,
Chairman.

The equivalent of the NBCE in the
U.S.

d) **Research Organizations**

i) *Foundation for Chiropractic
Education and Research* (FCER).
P.O. Box 4689, 704 East 4th Street,
Des Moines, IA 50306-4689 USA,
tel: 515-282-7118,
fax: 515-282-3347,
email: fcernow@aol.com.
Contacts: Deanna L. Beck, Director of
Administration, and Anthony L.
Rosner, PhD, Director of Research.
(Direct Boston line: 888-690-1378 or
617-734-3397.)

ii) *Consortial Center for Chiropractic
Research.*
c/o Palmer College of Chiropractic,
1000 Brady Street, Davenport, Iowa
52803, USA,
tel: 319-884-5162,
fax: 319-884-5227.
Contact: William Meeker, DC, MPH,
Chairman.

iii) *Consortium for Chiropractic Research in Canada*
c/o 1396 Eglinton Avenue West,
Toronto, Ontario M6C 2E4, Canada,
tel: 416-781-5656,
fax: 416-781-7344,
email: ccachiro@inforamp.net,
website: www.inforamp.net/
~ccachiro.
Contact: Allan Gotlib, DC, Research Programs Coordinator.

Participating institutions in this Consortium, established under the guidance of the Canadian Chiropractic Association, include the two chiropractic colleges in Canada, the universities of Calgary, Saskatchewan, Waterloo and York, and the Institute for Work and Health, Toronto.

e) **Professional Liability Insurance**.

i) *NCMIC Insurance Company* (NCMIC). 1452 29th Street, Suite 200, West Des Moines, Iowa 50266-1307, USA,
tel: 515-222-1736,
fax: 515-222-2951,
website: www.ncmic.com.
Contact: Mr. Larry Rister, Executive Vice-President, Louis Sportelli DC, President.

Chiropractors may obtain their professional liability/malpractice insurance from many private companies. One, established by the profession and by far the largest carrier for chiropractors in the U.S., is NCMIC.

ii) *Canadian Chiropractic Protective Association* (CCPA).
1396 Eglinton Avenue West,
Toronto, Ontario M6C 2E4, Canada,
tel: 416-781-5656,
fax: 416-781-7344,
email: ccachiro@inforamp.net,
website: www.inforamp.net/
~ccachiro.
Contact: Paul Carey DC, President.

The CCPA, modeled on the Canadian Medical Protective Association, is strictly speaking a mutual protective fund but, in lay terms, provides the equivalent of professional liability insurance. It is formally affiliated with the Canadian Chiropractic Association, and insures approximately 90% of Canada's chiropractors.

f) **Straights versus Mixers**. You may have heard the terms *straight chiropractors* and *mixers* used and, historically, this has been a significant internal conflict in the chiropractic profession in the U.S. That conflict has now been largely resolved. The distinctive feature of straight chiropractors was that they said it was neither their responsibility nor interest to perform a diagnosis. They only assessed and corrected spinal subluxations. They were not responsible for referral of a patient who might also need medical care. Accordingly they required a more limited scope of education.

In the 1970s and the 1980s there was a move to try to establish a second, straight level of chiropractic education, with its own colleges, accrediting agency and professional organizations. The straight chiropractic movement challenged the authority of the government-recognized accrediting agency, the CCE, in the courts but lost their final appeal in 1987. Many U.S. states have refused licensure to graduates of straight colleges. All chiropractic colleges now accept the one educational standard mandated by CCE.

Individual straight chiropractors also ran into legal problems. There is obvious inconsistency in having the right to deliver primary health care direct to patients, as chiropractors do, yet resisting the education and duty to perform a diagnosis. That point was made forcefully in the New Jersey Supreme Court case of *Rosenberg v Cahill*[1] in 1985 and a number of other cases.

The term *straight* is sometimes still used in a different and more informal sense— some chiropractors will say they have a *straight practice* meaning that they focus exclusively on spinal adjustment or manipulation without the use of adjunctive therapies such as TENS, ultrasound and other electrotherapies. However today there is no separate education, licensure, practice or professional organization for straight chiropractors.

C. Law

1. **Right to Practice.** Table 1 lists the countries in which the practice of chiropractic is recognized by governments and health authorities. Official recognition can be given in three different ways.

    a) **Legislation.** The first is by legislation, and there is now legislation to recognize and regulate the profession in Africa (e.g. Nigeria, South Africa and Zimbabwe), the Asian-Pacific region (e.g. Australia, Hong Kong, the Philippines and New Zealand), the Eastern Mediterranean (e.g. Cyprus, and Saudi Arabia), Europe (e.g. Belgium, Denmark, Finland, Norway, Sweden, Switzerland and the United Kingdom), Latin America (e.g. Mexico and Panama) and North America (Canada and the United States). In all instances legislation authorizes primary practice with the right and duty to diagnose, including the right to provide or order diagnostic imaging. (For details see Chapter 6, "Scope of Practice".) A more detailed review of the international legislation can be found in a paper titled *Legislative Approaches to the Regulation of the Chiropractic Profession.*[2]

    b) **General law.** Chiropractic practice may be recognized under general law without the existence of specific chiropractic legislation. This is the situation in many countries, for example Japan, which now has over 10,000 chiropractors (though not all educated to the international standard), The Netherlands with 150 chiropractors, and Trinidad & Tobago with five. Sometimes legality under general law has been confirmed by ministerial ruling, as for example in Fiji, Mauritius and Venezuela. On other occasions it has been confirmed by decisions of the courts, as in Brazil, Chile and Greece. Elsewhere there may be general legislation, as in Germany where chiropractors practice under umbrella legislation authorizing many types of health providers to practice natural health care methods under the general title of *heilpraktor*.

Table 1 Countries where Chiropractors are recognized by National Health Authorities

African Region	Eastern Mediterranean Region	European Region	North American Region
Botswana[a]	Cyprus[a]	Venezuela[b]	Bahamas[b]
Ethiopia[b]	Egypt[b]	**European Region**	Barbados[a]
Kenya[b]	Greece[b]	Belgium[a]	Belize[b]
Lesotho[a]	Israel[b]	Croatia[b]	Bermuda[b]
Mauritius[b]	Jordan[b]	Denmark[a]	British Virgin Islands[b]
Namibia[a]	Lebanon[b]	England[a]	Canada[a]
Nigeria[a]	Libya[b]	Finland[a]	Cayman Islands[b]
South Africa[a]	Morocco[b]	Germany[b]	Jamaica[b]
Swaziland[a]	Qatar[b]	Hungary[b]	Leeward Islands[a]
Zimbabwe[a]	Saudi Arabia[a]	Iceland[a]	Puerto Rico[a]
	Turkey[b]	Ireland[b]	Trinidad & Tobago[b]
Asian Region	United Arab Emirates[b]	Italy[c]	United States[a]
China-Hong Kong[a]		Liechtenstein[a]	US Virgin Islands[b]
Japan[b]		Netherlands[b]	
Malaysia[b]	**Latin American Region**	Norway[a]	
Philippines[a]	Argentina[b]	Portugal[c]	
Singapore[b]	Brazil[b]	Russian Federation[b]	
Taiwan[b]	Chile[b]	Slovakia[b]	
Thailand[c]	Columbia[b]	Sweden[a]	
	Costa Rica[b]	Switzerland[a]	
Pacific Region	Ecuador[b]		
Australia[a]	Guatemala[b]		
Fiji[b]	Honduras[b]		
Guam[a]	Mexico[a]		
New Caledonia[b]	Panama[a]		
New Zealand[a]	Peru[b]		
Papua New Guinea[b]			

Note: Listed according to the seven world regions adopted by the World Federation of Chiropractic. In most other countries there are no chiropractors in practice, and national health authorities have not considered recognition or lack of recognition.

Legend:
[a] Recognized pursuant to legislation.
[b] Recognized pursuant to general law.
[c] *De facto* recognition.

c) **De facto acceptance**. This is a third method of recognition, and applies in countries where the practice of chiropractic is technically in breach of medical practice law, but is acknowledged and not obstructed by national health authorities. This is possible because chiropractic practice is non-invasive, makes no use of drugs or surgery and is recognized to be of public benefit. In Italy, for example, the practice of chiropractic remains technically illegal. However the government and health authorities have acknowledged the value of qualified chiropractic services, the government actually pays for them in some clinical settings and Italy's 200 chiropractors no longer face the threat of prosecutions.

The five countries that have taken legal action against duly qualified chiropractors in recent years are France, Iran, South Korea, Spain and Thailand. Paradoxically, chiropractors in these countries experience significant medical referral of patients who include senior legislators and many medical practitioners.

2. **Professional Titles**. Various titles are authorized by law in different countries. The title *chiropractor* or its equivalent (e.g. *chiropraktor* (Ger), *chiropraticien(ne)* (Fr), *kiropraktor* (Scand), *quiropraxia* (Sp)) is universal. Use of the title *doctor of chiropractic* is common throughout North America. This reflects the fact that in North America the title *doctor* is used by all primary contact health professionals with the right and duty to diagnose, including dentists, optometrists, osteopaths, podiatrists and psychologists. Many states in the U.S. also authorize use of the title *chiropractic physician*. These states, which include for example California, Florida, Illinois, New York and Ohio,

---

CAP. 428   *Chiropractors Registration*   第428章   脊醫註冊條例   3

CHAPTER 428

CHIROPRACTORS REGISTRATION

An Ordinance to provide for the registration of chiropractors namely, persons trained and qualified in the practice of chiropractic including the practice of the prevention, diagnosis and treatment of functional disorders of the human body through manipulation of the joints, particularly of the vertebral column and peripheral joints, including the pelvis; the disciplinary control of the professional activities of registered chiropractors; and for matters related to such registration and disciplinary control.

第428章

脊醫註冊條例

本條例旨在對脊醫(即在脊骨療法專業及其中所包括的藉矯正關節(尤指脊椎及周圍關節,亦包括骨盆)的方法對人體機能失調的病症加以預防並作出診斷治療的專業方面曾接受訓練並符合資格的人)的註冊、註冊脊醫專業事務的紀律管制與該等註冊及紀律管制有關的事宜作出規定。

ELIZABETH II   c. 17

Chiropractors Act 1994

1994 CHAPTER 17

An Act to establish a body to be known as the General Chiropractic Council; to provide for the regulation of the chiropractic profession, including making provision as to the registration of chiropractors and as to their professional education and conduct; to make provision in connection with the development and promotion of the profession; to amend, and make provision in connection with, the Osteopaths Act 1993; and for connected purposes.   [5th July 1994]

ΠΑΡΑΡΤΗΜΑ ΠΡΩΤΟ
ΤΗΣ ΕΠΙΣΗΜΗΣ ΕΦΗΜΕΡΙΔΑΣ ΤΗΣ ΔΗΜΟΚΡΑΤΙΑΣ
Αρ. 2584 της 22ας ΜΑΡΤΙΟΥ 1991
ΝΟΜΟΘΕΣΙΑ

Ο περί Εγγραφής Χειροπρακτών Νόμος του 1991 εκδίδεται με δημοσίευση στην Επίσημη Εφημερίδα της Κυπριακής Δημοκρατίας σύμφωνα με το Άρθρο 52 του Συντάγματος.

Αριθμός 62 του 1991
ΝΟΜΟΣ ΠΟΥ ΠΡΟΝΟΕΙ ΓΙΑ ΤΗΝ ΕΓΓΡΑΦΗ ΧΕΙΡΟΠΡΑΚΤΩΝ ΚΑΙ ΓΙΑ ΣΥΝΑΦΗ ΘΕΜΑΤΑ
Η Βουλή των Αντιπροσώπων ψηφίζει ως ακολούθως:

1. Ο παρών Νόμος θα αναφέρεται ως ο περί Εγγραφής Χειροπρακτών   Συνοπτικός Νόμος του 1991.   τίτλος.
2. Στον παρόντα Νόμο—   Ερμηνεία.
«Έφορος» σημαίνει τον Έφορο που ορίζεται με βάση το άρθρο 3·
«Μητρώο» σημαίνει το Μητρώο Εγγραφής Χειροπρακτών που προβλέπεται από το άρθρο 4·
«Υπουργός» σημαίνει τον Υπουργό Υγείας·
«χειροπράκτης» σημαίνει το πρόσωπο το οποίο ασκεί τη χειροπρακτική·

Chiropractic laws exist not only in all U.S. states, but in many other countries. Here are extracts from the Hong Kong Chiropractors' Legislation Ordinance, 1992; the U.K. Chiropractors' Act, 1994, and the Chiropractors' Act 1991 in Cyprus.

recognize three categories of physicians—chiropractic, medical and osteopathic.

The degree granted by chiropractic colleges is a doctor of chiropractic degree. This means that in *Joanna Smith, DC,* the initials refer to both a professional qualification and professional title.

One major reason for legislation to regulate a health profession is to prevent unqualified practitioners or lay persons from passing themselves off as members of that profession, exposing the public to ineffective or harmful treatments. For this reason chiropractic laws typically prohibit persons without a license from using the above protected titles or otherwise holding themselves out expressly or by implication as being engaged in the practice of chiropractic.

3. **Scope of Practice**. This is discussed in a separate chapter—see Chapter 6, "Scope of Practice".

4. **Licensing Boards and Regulation.** Typically the licensing board, as for medicine and other licensed health care professions, adopts a model of self-regulation with a mix of chiropractors and lay members. The U.S. states with the most licensed chiropractors—California with approximately 10,000 and Florida with over 4,000 chiropractors—have licensing boards with 7 members—5 chiropractors and 2 lay persons. All members are appointed by government. Montana, with 360 chiropractors, and Nebraska, with 250, each has an appointed board with 3 chiropractors and 1 lay person.

Canadian regulatory boards tend to be larger, with professional members elected rather than appointed by government. The province of Ontario, with approximately 2,000 chiropractors, has a licensing board of 16 persons—9 being chiropractors elected by the profession and 7 lay persons appointed by government.

Sometimes the chiropractic licensing board functions under the umbrella of an interdisciplinary board. In the State of Illinois, with 2,500 chiropractors, there is a Medical Licensing Board (MLB) which coordinates regulation of the three categories of health providers defined as physicians in that state—chiropractic, medical and osteopathic physicians. The MLB has 7 members—5 medical doctors, 1 chiropractic doc-

tor and 1 osteopathic doctor. However, day-to-day licensing and disciplinary functions for each profession are handled by separate subsidiary boards.

The functions of all these licensing boards are to regulate the profession in the public interest—hold examinations for licensure, provide ongoing rules and regulations and, for the practice of the profession, respond to public inquiries and complaints, take disciplinary action to suspend the license of or otherwise penalize chiropractors guilty of unprofessional behavior or otherwise breaching licensing laws, monitor continuing education, etc. For further details see Chapter 4, "Education and Licensure."

D. Education

Chiropractic education is much more regulated and extensive than most people appreciate. For a full discussion see Chapter 4.

E. Literature and Research

1. **Literature**. Until the 1980s chiropractic literature was not strong. However, after 20 years of quite dramatic growth in academic writing and research, the profession now has an established literature base, both in its own periodicals and text books and in other medical and health science publications.

a) **Text Books**. More major texts have been published in the last 10 years than in the previous history of the profession and many are of the highest quality by any standards.

  • The first edition of Foreman and Croft's *Whiplash Injuries: The Cervical Acceleration/Deceleration Syndrome*, when published in 1988, was described by Ruth Jackson, MD, a leading medical author in that field, as "the most remarkable compilation of scientific and factual data thus far published concerning the many facets of the cervical spine."[3]

  • The second edition of *Essentials of Skeletal Radiology* (1996),[4] by chiropractic radiologists Yochum and Rowe, was glowingly reviewed in the *New England Journal of Medicine* as a "textbook that should be required reading for any student of radiology . . . This textbook is indeed special and will serve as a reference for the development of skeletal radiology for succeeding generations."[5]

- Another major chiropractic radiology text *Clinical Imaging: With Skeletal Chest and Abdomen Pattern Differentials* (1999),[6] edited by Marchiori has contributions from many chiropractic and medical radiologists. It is praised as "an outstanding text" from "an outstanding group of radiologists" by Francis Burgener, MD, Professor of Radiology, University of Rochester Medical Center, Rochester, New York, in his foreword.

  Professor Vert Mooney, Past-Chairman, Department of Orthopedic Surgery, University of California at San Diego, in a foreword in *Spinal Rehabilitation*,[7] edited by Stude of the Northwestern College of Chiropractic, says that the text "clearly demonstrates the ongoing integration of chiropractic into comprehensive medical care", is "a unique blend of the two major physical approaches to spinal care—manual therapy and active exercise", and "is the way of the future" and "foward thinking at its very best".

- *Chiropractic Technique* (1993) by Bergmann, Petersen and Lawrence,[8] *Chiropractic Manipulative Skills* (1996) by Byfield[9] and *Mechanically Assisted Manual Techniques: Distraction Procedures* by Bergmann and Davis (1998)[10] are examples of sophisticated texts on techniques of chiropractic manipulation and mobilization.

  A major chiropractic text on soft-tissue examination and treatment is *Functional Soft-tissue Examination and Treatment of Manual Methods*,[11] edited by Hammer. This and texts such as *Principles and Practice of Chiropractic* (1992) edited by Haldeman,[12] *Rehabilitation of the Spine: A Practitioner's Manual* (1996) edited by Liebenson,[13] the already mentioned *Spinal Rehabilitation* (1999) edited by Stude,[7] and *Conservative Management of Cervical Spine Syndromes* (1999) edited by Murphy,[14] draw together contributions from

leading experts from many disciplines worldwide in a way that was not possible in the past.

- *Fundamentals of Chiropractic Diagnosis and Management* (1991) edited by Lawrence[15] and *Differential Diagnosis for the Chiropractor: Protocols and Algorithms* (1997) by Souza[16] are major general clinical texts of 600 and 750 pages respectively.

- There are texts of similar quality in many specialty areas such as:

  Anatomy (e.g. *Basic and Clinical Anatomy of the Spine, Spinal Cord and ANS*, 1996, Cramer and Darby[17]);

  Back disorders (*Clinical Anatomy and Management of Low-Back Pain*, 1997, edited by Giles and Singer[18]);

  Cervical spine disorders (*Upper Cervical Syndrome: Chiropractic Diagnosis and Treatment*, 1988, edited by Vernon[19]); *Whiplash Injuries: The Cervical Acceleration/Deceleration Syndrome*, 1988 by Foreman and Croft[3] and *Conservative Management of Cervical Spine Syndromes*, 1999, edited by Murphy.[14]);

  Head pain (*Chiropractic Approach to Head Pain*, 1994, edited by Curl[20]);

  Pediatrics (*Pediatric Chiropractic*, 1999, edited by Anrig and Plaugher[21]);

  Sports injuries (*Sports Injuries of the Shoulder: Conservative Management*, 1994, edited by Souza[22] and *Conservative Management of Sports Injuries*, 1998, edited by Hyde and Gengenbach.[23])

  Lynton Giles, DC, PhD and Kevin Singer, PT, PhD, prominent researchers from Australia, are a chiropractor and a physiotherapist respectively. Their excellent text on low-back pain has contributions from world-renowned authors from the professions of chiropractic, medicine, osteopathy, physiotherapy and psychology. They are listed in Table 2. This text, published by a leading British health science publisher, Butterworth-Heinemann, is designed for use in educational programs for all

Table 2 Contributors— Giles & Singer Text

Harold S. Amonoo-Kuofi, MB, ChB, PhD, Professor of Clinical Anatomy, Department of Anatomy, College of Medicine and King Khalid University Hospital, Riyadh, Saudi Arabia.

Mohammed G.Y. El-Badawi, MB, BCh, MS, MD, Professor Anatomy, College of Medicine, Suez Canal University, Ismailia, Egypt

Kim Burton, PhD, DO, MERgS, Director, Spinal Research Unit, University of Huddersfield, UK

S.H. Burns, DC, FCCS(C), Private Practice of Chiropractic, Saskatoon, Saskatchewan, Canada

Robert Clarke, DO, Associate Osteopath and Research Associate, Spinal Research Unit, University of Huddersfield, UK

Colin M. Crawford, BAppSc(Chiro), GradDip (Neurosci), FCCS(C), Research Fellow, James Cook University of North Queensland, Townsville, Australia

Henry Vernon Crock, MD, MS, FRCS, FRACS, Honorary Senior Lecturer, Orthopaedic Department, Royal Post Graduate Medical School, Hammersmith Hospital, London

Stephen J. Edmondston, Dip PT, Adv Dip PT, PhD, Lecturer, School of Physiotherapy, Curtin University, Perth WA, Australia

Robert L. Elvey, BAppSc, PGDipMT, Senior Lecturer, School of Physiotherapy, Curtin University, Perth WA, Australia

Lynton Giles, MSc, DC, PhD, Chief Executive Director and Research Director, National Centre for Multidisciplinary Studies of Back Pain, Townsville General Hospital, Townsville, Queensland, Australia

Mats Grönblad, MD, PhD, Associate Professor and Senior Lecturer in Physical Medicine and Rehabilitation, University of Helsinki, Finland

Basil James, BSc, MBBCh, FRANZCP, FRACP, FRSPsych, Professor of Psychiatry and Behavioural Sciences, Queensland, Australia

J. Randy Jinkins, MD, FACR, Director of Neuroradiology, University of Texas Health Science Center, San Antonio, Texas, USA

Shinichi Kikuchi, MD, PhD, Professor and Chairman, Department of Orthopaedic Surgery, Fukushima City, Japan

Bruce R. Knolmayer, MD, Department of Orthopedics, Georgetown University Medical Center, USA

Robert McAlindon, MD, Department of Orthopedics, Georgetown University Medical Center, USA

Tim McClune, DO, Associate Osteopath and Research Associate, Spinal Research Unit, University of Huddersfield, UK

Frank McDonald, Clinical Psychologist, Department of Psychiatry, Townsville General Hospital, Townsville, Queensland, Australia

Dale R. Mierau, BSPE, DC, MSc(Orth), FCCS(C), Private Practice of Chiropractic, Saskatoon, Saskatchewan, Canada

K.P. Singer, MSc, PT, PhD, Associate Professor, School of Physiotherapy, Curtin University of Technology, Shenton Park, Western Australia, Australia

Three of the profession's scientific journals are shown —*Topics in Clinical Chiropractic* (Aspen); *The Journal of Manipulative and Physiological Therapeutics* (Mosby); and *Journal of the Neuromusculoskeletal System* (Data Trace for the American Chiropractic Association).

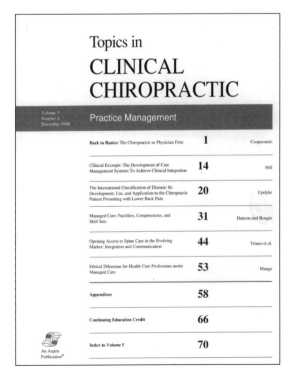

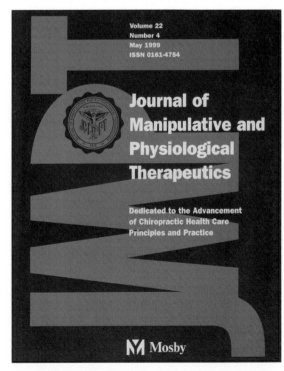

the above professions. The foreword is by Professor John Frymoyer, Dean of Medicine, University of Vermont, who praises the text and the fact that it is "built around the basic model of interdisciplinary collaboration."

- *Managing Low-Back Pain* (1992, 3rd edition) edited by Kirkaldy-Willis, a Canadian orthopedic surgeon and Burton, an American neurosurgeon, is an example of a leading medical text on back pain in which the principal authors of the chapter on manipulation are chiropractors, Cassidy and Thiel.[24] Other major medical texts with similar chapters by chiropractors are Melzack and Wall's *Textbook of Pain*,[25] Frymoyer's *The Adult Spine*,[26] and Hochschuler's *Treat Your Back Without Surgery: The Best Non-Surgical Alternatives to Eliminating Back and Neck Pain*.[27]

b) **Periodicals.** Periodicals include journals, such as the chiropractic profession's leading peer-reviewed indexed journal titled *The Journal of Manipulative and Physiological Therapeutics (JMPT)* which has been published in the United States since 1978, and series. Series include texts that are published annually and in chiropractic include *Advances in Chiropractic* and the *Year Book of Chiropractic*, both published by Mosby in the U.S.A.

c) **Scientific Journals**. Peer-reviewed chiropractic journals for the publication of original research are:

Table 3 **Editorial Board—JMPT**

Alan H. Adams, DC, MS – *Whittier, California*
Delmas J. Allen, PhD – *Whittier, California*
Gil C. Allen, DC, PhD – *Glen Head, New York*
William Assendelft, MD, PhD – *Amsterdam, The Netherlands*
Alan C. Breen, DC, PhD – *Bournemouth, England*
Patricia C. Brennan, PhD – *Lombard, Illinois*
J. David Cassidy, DC, PhD – *Saskatoon, Saskatchewan, Canada*
Keith Charlton, DC – *Oxford, England*
James M. Cox, DC – *Fort Wayne, Indiana*
Jeffrey R. Cram, PhD – *Nevada City, California*
Vaclav Dvorak, MD – *Bonaduz, Switzerland*
Phillip Ebrall, BAppSc (Chiro) – *Bundoora, Australia*
L.G.F. Giles, DC, PhD – *Queensland, Australia*
Phillip E. Greenman, DO – *East Lansing, Michigan*
Mitchell Haas, DC – *Portland, Oregon*
Scott Haldeman, DC, MD, PhD – *Santa Ana, California*
Daniel Hansen, DC – *Olympia, Washington*
Cheryl Hawk, DC, PhD – *Davenport, Iowa*
Walter Herzog, PhD – *Calgary, Alberta, Canada*
Maria A. Hondras, DC, MPH – *Portland, Oregon*
Jennifer R. Jamison, MBBCh, PhD, EdD – *Bundoora, Australia*
Vladimir Janda, Doc, MUDr – *Prague, Czech Republic*
Robert Jansen, PhD – *San Jose, California*
Joseph C. Keating, Jr. PhD – *Whittier, California*
Andries M. Kleynhans, DC – *Bundoora, Victoria, Australia*
Irvin M. Korr, PhD – *Boulder , Colorado*
Charlotte Leboeuf-Yde, DC, MPH, PhD – *Odense, Denmark*
Karel Lewit, MUDr, Doc, DSc – *Prague, Czech Republic*
Marion McGregor-Triano, DC, MSc – *Richardson, Texas*
William C. Meeker, DC, MPH – *San Jose, California*
Robert Mootz, DC – *Olympia, Washington*
D. Dale Nansel, PhD – *San Jose, California*
Niels Grunnet-Nilsson, DC, MD, PhD – *Odense, Denmark*
Joanne Nyiendo, PhD – *Portland, Oregon*
David H. Peterson, DC – *Portland, Oregon*
Reed B. Phillips, DC, PhD – *Whittier, California*
Anthony L. Rosner, PhD – *Brookline, Massachusetts*
Akio Sato, MD, PhD – *Tokyo, Japan*
Charles Sawyer, DC – *Bloomington, Minnesota*
Gary Schultz, DC – *Whittier, California*
Robert C. Shiel, PhD – *Lombard, Illinois*
John J. Triano, DC, PhD – *Plano, Texas*
Howard T. Vernon, DC, FCCS – *Toronto, Ontario, Canada*
Walter I. Wardwell, PhD – *Storrs, Connecticut*
Terry R. Yochum, DC, DACBR – *Denver, Colorado*

JNMS
Journal of the Neuromusculoskeletal System

A Journal of the American Chiropractic Association

VOLUME 6, NUMBER 2   SUMMER 1998   ISSN 1067-8239

Data Trace Publishing Company

General

Australia: *Chiropractic Journal of Australia*. Publisher: Chiropractors' Association of Australia, Sydney.

Canada: *Journal of the Canadian Chiropractic Association*. Publisher: Canadian Chiropractic Association, Toronto.

Europe: *European Journal of Chiropractic*. Publisher: Blackwell, Oxford (for the European Chiropractors' Union).

Japan: *Japanese Journal of Chiropractic Sciences*. Publisher: Japanese Chiropractic Association, Tokyo.

U.S.A.: *Journal of Manipulative and Physiological Therapeutics*. Publisher: Mosby Yearbook, St. Louis, Missouri (for the National College of Chiropractic).

U.S.A.: *Journal of the Neuromusculo-skeletal System*. Publisher: Data Trace, Baltimore, Maryland (for the American Chiropractic Association, Arlington, Virginia).

U.S.A.: *Topics in Clinical Chiropractic*. Publisher: Aspen Publishers, Gaithersburg, Maryland.

U.S.A.: *Chiropractic Research Journal*. Publisher: Life University, Marietta, Georgia.

Special Interest

U.S.A.: *Chiropractic History*. Publisher: Association for the History of Chiropractic, Davenport, Iowa.

U.S.A.: *Chiropractic Technique*. Publisher: Lippincott Williams and Wilkins, Baltimore, Maryland, (for the National College of Chiropractic).

Table 4 Editorial Board, JNMS

EDITOR-IN-CHIEF
Scott Haldeman, DC, MD, PhD
University of California, Irvine

EDITOR	**SPECIAL FEATURES EDITOR**
William C. Meeker, DC, MPH	Rand S. Swenson, DC, MD, PhD
Palmer Center for Chiropractic Research	Dartmouth-Hitchcock Medical Center
Davenport, Iowa	Lebanon, New Hampshire

SECTION EDITORS

Biochemistry & Nutrition	Epidemiology & Public Health	Physical Therapy
Anthony Rosner, PhD	*Reed Phillips, DC, DACBR, PhD*	*Anthony Delitto, PT, PhD*
Bioethics & Humanities	Manual & Manipulative Therapy/	Physiology
Dana J. Lawrence, DC	Osteopathy	*Akio Sato, MD, PhD*
Biomechanics & Ergonomics	*Phillip Greenman, DO*	Psychology and Behavioral Medicine
M.R. Gudavalli, PhD	Medical Imaging	*Nelson Hendler, MSc, MD*
Chiropractic Sciences	*Charles Aprill, MD*	Radiology & Imaging
J. David Cassidy, DC, PhD	Orthopedics	*Terry R. Yochum, DC, DACBR*
Clinical Anatomy	*Hamilton Hall, MD*	Sports Injuries & Exercise Injury
Gregory D. Cramer, DC, PhD	Physical Medicine & Rehabilitation	*Thomas E. Hyde, DC, DACBSP*
	Michael S. Kaplan, MD, PhD	

ASSOCIATE EDITORS

Alan H. Adams, DC, DACBN	Gary M. Guebert, DC, DACBR	Gary D. Schultz, DC, DACBR
Michael S. Barry, DC, DACBR	Kevin R. Gurr, MD	Lawrence Timothy Sellers, DC,
Kathleen Baumgardner, DC, CCSP	Scott L. Havsy, DO, DAAPM	DACBR
Pat Brennan, PhD	Walter Herzog, PhD	Dennis Skogsbergh, DC, DABCO,
Raymond R. Brodeur, DC, PhD	Joseph W. Howe, DC, DACBR	DACBR
James E. Carter, DC, DACBR	Sharon A. Jaeger, DC, DACBR	Monica Smith, DC, PhD
Raymond N. Conley, DC, DACBR	Russel Jaffe, MD, PhD	Tilden H. Sokoloff, MSc, DC,
Arthur C. Croft, DC, MS, DABCO	Norman W. Kettner, DC, DACBR	FCCS(C)
John Danchik, PhD	Partap S. Khalsa, DC, PhD, FACO	Haymo Thiel, MSc, DC, FCCS(C)
Richard E. Erhard, PT, DC	William E. Litterer, MSc, DC, DACBR	Howard Vernon, DC, FCCS(C)
Ronald Evans, DC, FACO	Dale Mierau, MSc, DC, FCCS(C)	David Wickes, DC
Marianne Gengenbach, DC, CCSP	Silvano A. Mior, DC, FCCS(C)	Steven L. Wolf, PhD, FAPTA

U.S.A.: *Journal of the Chiropractic Humanities*. Publisher: National College of Chiropractic, Lombard, Illinois.

U.S.A.: *Journal of Sports Chiropractic and Rehabilitation*. Publisher: Lippincott Williams and Wilkins, Baltimore, Maryland.

U.S.A.: *Topics in Diagnostic Radiology and Advanced Imaging*. Publisher: American Chiropractic Association Council on Diagnostic Imaging, Palatine, Illinois.

Editorial Boards

Tables 3 and 4 give the editorial boards of the two leading journals—the *Journal of Manipulative and Physiological Therapeutics (JMPT)* which has been published since 1978 and is indexed in Index Medicus, and the *Journal of the Neuromusculoskeletal System (JNMS)* which has been published since 1993 and is indexed in the Cumulative Index to Nursing and Allied Health Literature (CINAHL). Both editorial boards are international, multidisciplinary and include prominent researchers from the medical, osteopathic and physical therapy scientific communities. Many of the chiropractic board members have basic science doctorates, medical degrees and other postgraduate qualifications such as masters degrees in public health.

Content

Most of the papers published in the chiropractic literature, not surprisingly, come from chiropractors and chiropractic research institutions. However research is routinely received from other disciplines. Table 5 gives the table of contents to the December 1998 issue of JMPT. You will see papers from:

- A chiropractic and medical research team in Japan

- A chiropractic and medical research team in Denmark

- Physiotherapy researchers from Australia

- Chiropractors from Australia

- Basic scientists from China

- A basic sciences and medical research team from France

Similarly chiropractic research is now regularly published in leading medical journals, such as the *Annals of Internal Medicine, British Medical Journal, Clinical Biomechanics, Journal of the American Medical Association, New England Journal of Medicine, Pain* and *Spine*.

2. **Chiropractic Research**. Up until the 1980s the chiropractic profession failed to produce a reasonable volume of research. Chiropractors could give a number of credible reasons—such as major trial design problems which resulted in little clinical research in

By 1993 the British Medical Association was citing the chiropractic profession as the best example of a newer profession that was conducting good quality clinical research to establish its safety and effectiveness.

physical medicine generally, complete exclusion from public facilities and funding and the financial priorities of ensuring the legal right to practice and upgrading undergraduate education. But the reality is there was little research effort.

By the 1980s that had changed. In 1986 an Australian federal government Medicare Benefits Review Committee, reviewing chiropractic with a view to funding of chiropractic services, noted the "significant shift in the last decade in attitude towards the issue of scientific research" and dismissed medical criticisms of chiropractic research as "something of a red herring."[28] By 1993 the British Medical Association was citing the chiropractic profession as the best example of a newer profession that was conducting good quality clinical research to establish its safety and effectiveness.[29]

a) **Organizations**. Significant new organizations in North America are:

i) **Consortial Center for Chiropractic Research**—United States (Director, William Meeker, DC, MPH, Palmer Center for Chiropractic Research, 1000 Brady Street, Davenport, Iowa, 52803, USA, tel: 319-884-5000 fax: 319-326-9897). This organization, formed with the guidance and support of the federal government, includes research representatives from government, chiropractic colleges and university faculties of medicine and other health sciences. Its two main functions are to bring an interdisciplinary leadership group together annually at a national workshop to establish a chiropractic research agenda, and to attract public and private research funds to chiropractic research projects that have the greatest priority and importance.

The annual workshops, which began in 1996, are financed by the Bureau of Health Professions, Health Resources and Services Administration, U.S. Department of Health and Human Services (HRSA). In the six months following the 1997 meeting,

for example, U.S. federal agencies made these research grants totaling $4.3 million dollars:

- *Consortial Center for Chiropractic Research*—$2.6 million (Center for Alternative Medicine, National Institutes of Health).

- *Low-Back Pain: Long Term Outcome and Practice Activities*, Mitchell Haas, DC, Western States Chiropractic College— $960,697 (HRSA).

- *Spinal Manipulation Versus Mobilization for Neck Pain*, Hal Morgenstern, PhD, UCLA/Los

Table 5 Table of Contents—JMPT December 1998

Angeles College of Chiropractic—$854,464.

- *Flexion Distraction Versus Medical Care for Low-Back Pain,* Ram Gudavalli, PhD, Texas Back Institute—$439,661.

Two things about these grants are noteworthy. Firstly, although they are very modest amounts compared with government-funded medical research (which totaled at least $13.2 billion in 1997) they represent more than total previous government funding for chiropractic research. Secondly, each of the specific research projects that attracted government funding follows pilot or preliminary studies performed and funded by the chiropractic profession.

ii) **Consortium for Chiropractic Research—Canada**. This has a similar role to the U.S. consortium but was established by the Canadian Chiropractic Association without government funding or assistance. Participating institutions include both of the Canadian chiropractic colleges (Canadian Memorial Chiropractic College, Toronto, and the School of Chiropractic, University of Quebec, Trois Rivières), the Institute of Work and Health, which is affiliated with the University of Toronto, and the universities of Calgary, Saskatchewan, Waterloo and York.

The first government funding attracted by the Consortium is a Government of Ontario grant of $1 million to Howard Vernon, DC, (Canadian Memorial Chiropractic College) and Gwen Jansz, MD (University of Toronto) for a randomized controlled trial comparing chiropractic, medical and chiropractic/medical combined management of patients with chronic tension-type headache.

iii) **Foundation for Chiropractic Education and Research**. (Deanna L. Beck, Director of Administration, P.O. Box 4689, 704 East 4th Street, Des Moines, Iowa, 50306-4689 USA, tel: 515-282-7118, fax: 515-282-3347, email: fcernow@aol.com. Director of Research: Anthony L. Rosner, PhD.) Since the early 1980s a number of private research foundations have been established by chiropractors in private practice wishing to support research. These include the Foundation for Advancement of Chiropractic Education (FACE), established by U.S. practitioner Dr. William Harris in 1981 (which has since contributed more than $3 million principally to building research infrastructure at chiropractic colleges), and the National Institute of Chiropractic Research (NICR), established by U.S. practitioner Dr. Arlan Fuhr in 1987 (which has now contributed more than $1 million to specific clinical research projects.) Sixteen U.S. chiropractic colleges established the Consortium for Chiropractic Research (CCR) in 1989.

However the chiropractic profession's most senior and established research organization is the Foundation for Chiropractic Education and Research (FCER) established in 1944. By 1990 the annual budget of FCER, based largely on contributions from individual chiropractors and chiropractic-related businesses, was about $2 million. Major additional funding in recent years has come from the NCMIC Insurance Company.

b) **Research Conferences**. The two principal forums for presentation of original chiropractic research are:

- The biennial Scientific Symposium of the World Federation of Chiropractic (WFC).

- The International Conference on Spinal Manipulation (ICSM), which is the annual meeting of the Foundation for Chiropractic Education and Research.

Chiropractic researchers, often now working in multidisciplinary research teams, also regularly present their work at predominantly medical or interdisciplinary annual meetings such as those of the American Back Society, American Public Health Association, European Spine Society, International Society for

Study of the Lumbar Spine, North American Cervicogenic Headache Society, North American Primary Care Research Group and North American Spine Society.

c) **Scope of Research**. As the above review of chiropractic literature illustrates, there are now well-qualified chiropractors throughout the world producing a steady volume of research in both the basic and clinical sciences. This research, referred to in more detail in various sections of this book, includes studies of:

Recent research confirms precise forces of manipulation at the joint surface are significantly influenced by type of technique and by patient posture.

i) Anatomy—for examples see Chapter 1, page 5.

ii) How manipulation works and its documented immediate effects—see Chapter 7, page 102.

iii) Back pain—safety and effectiveness, cost-effectiveness, patient satisfaction—see Chapter 8, pages 107–121.

iv) Neck pain and headache—Chapter 6, pages 71–75.

v) Other conditions—Chapter 6, pages 76–88.

vi) Epidemiology. For example, who uses chiropractic services (95% have musculoskeletal pain including headache—see the recent study by Hurwitz et al. in the *American Journal of Public Health*[30]), and how common back pain and spinal dysfunction are in teenage children (see studies by Cassidy, Mierau et al. in Canada[31] and Leboeuf-Yde et al. in Denmark.[32] It is much more common than you might think—the large Danish survey [29,424 persons] finds that the steepest increase in the first episode of back pain is for adolescent boys and girls aged 12–14, and that over 50% of young women have had back pain by age 18, 50% of young men by age 20).

vii) Basic sciences (e.g. molecular research, biomechanical research). Many interesting areas of research

could be discussed. You might expect for example, that one thing being measured by chiropractic researchers would be the precise body forces generated by chiropractors using different chiropractic techniques. Some people express the view that forces are inadequate to produce real effects, others have said forces are too great and could be dangerous. Detailed research is being done in a number of centers, by chiropractors and biomechanical engineers such as Walter Herzog, PhD, Gregory Kawchuk, DC, and Philip Conway, DC, at the University of Calgary in Canada, John Triano, DC, PhD, and Albert Schultz, PhD, at the Texas Back Institute and University of Michigan and Ram Gudavalli, PhD, at the National College of Chiropractic.

This work assesses not only forces where the doctor's hand meets the patient's body, but also forces internally at the joint surfaces. Recent research by Triano and Schultz studying 6 chiropractors using 3 different techniques each on 11 patients confirms:

- Precise forces of manipulation at the joint surface are significantly influenced by type of technique and by patient posture.

- Clinically significant forces are delivered at the joint surface level.

- These forces are "similar to those observed in common daily tasks on jobs requiring lifting and twisting movements."[33]

F. **Funding for Chiropractic Services.**

The degree to which there is government and private third party payment for chiropractic services constantly changes according to time and jurisdiction so this section provides a summary overview only.

1. **Government Funding**. Over the past 20 years four government commissions in Australia (1986),[34] New Zealand (1978),[35] Sweden (1987)[36] and Ontario, Canada (1993),[37] have been asked to study and report on whether there should be government fund-

ing for chiropractic services—all have said yes. This has led to varying degrees of coverage in Australia (veterans only), Canada (part funding for all patients in most provinces) and Sweden (part funding for all patients in approximately one-third of the health regions).

There is also government funding in Denmark (nationally for all patients), Israel (nationally through health maintenance organizations for all patients), Italy (only on medical referral in designated interdisciplinary clinics), Norway (nationally for all patients), Switzerland (in all cantons and federally—Switzerland was the first country to establish government funding for chiropractic services), the U.K. (for patients receiving chiropractic services through National Health Service contracts held by groups of general practitioners who include chiropractic services in their plan) and the U.S. (for seniors under Medicare, for the disadvantaged under Medicaid, and since 1995, to the U.S. military and their families at 13 bases throughout the U.S. as part of a pilot project for integration of chiropractic services throughout the U.S. military health care system).

2. **Workers' Compensation and Automobile Insurance**. These plans typically include coverage of chiropractic services on a similar basis to medical services in the U.S. states, Canadian provinces, Australian states and several European countries.

3. **Employee Benefits Plans**. Private insurance coverage under employee benefit plans has become available wherever the profession has become established. In the U.S. over 80% of employees in conventional insurance plans, preferred provider organizations (PPOs) and point of service plans have full or partial coverage for chiropractic services,[38] but the figure is currently less for health maintenance organizations (HMOs).

China-Hong Kong only has 50 chiropractors and the profession has only been licensed by law since 1994 but a majority of employees have coverage for chiropractic services. Mauritius, an island country in the Indian Ocean, provides a colorful example. Dr. Rajinder Roy became the first chiropractor to establish a practice in Mauritius in 1994. Shortly thereafter insurers began referring

to him back pain patients who were scheduled to be flown to South Africa for back surgery. Surgery was not needed in the first 20 consecutive cases and, as a result, many insurers now provide third party funding for his services.[39]

4. **U.S.—Sources of Reimbursement**. The U.S. health care system is in an era of constant and rapid change. From 1963 45 states (all except Hawaii, Idaho, Oregon, Vermont and Wyoming) passed state law mandates for chiropractic benefits—typically requiring health insurers offering conventional group fee-for-service policies to include chiropractic services. Then, however, came the rise of managed care and health maintenance organizations which were exempted from these state laws. Initially the coverage of chiropractic services in HMOs, as with all services seen as specialist services by gatekeepers and their managers, were heavily restricted. Now coverage is increasing.

On the overall question of sources of payment for chiropractic services—how much is paid by the patient and how much by different third party payers—studies by the American Chiropractic Association[40] and the RAND Corporation[30] are fairly consistent and, read together, report the following sources of payment in the early 1990s:

Patient—out-of-pocket	25%
Private insurance—	
employee benefits, indemnity	33%
Auto insurance	12%
Workers' compensation	10%
Medicare and Medicaid	10%
Managed care	10%
	100%

Table 6 (page 43) lists the detailed results of the RAND study, which applies to the years 1985–1991, and the ACA survey, which applies to the year 1995. These show a trend away from private indemnity insurance (dropping from 41.8% in the late 1980s to 28.6% in 1995) and towards managed care (rising from 3.7% to 8.6%). Because managed care was slow to fund chiropractic services, direct payments from patients increased over this period.

A 1993 KMPG Peat Marwick/Wayne State University survey of 1,953 employers across the U.S. representing 68.8 million workers, summarized in Table 7, reported that:

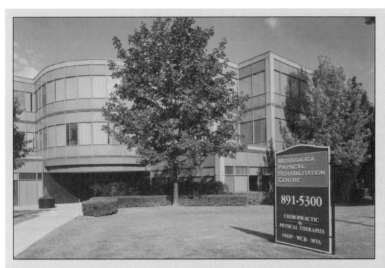

At the Mississauga Physical Rehabilitation Centre in Toronto, a chiropractic rehabilitation facility that is also a government-designated assessment center for motor vehicle injuries, chiropractor Dr. Carlan Stants reviews imaging studies with staff, and a patient is assessed for functional abilities and fitness to return to work.

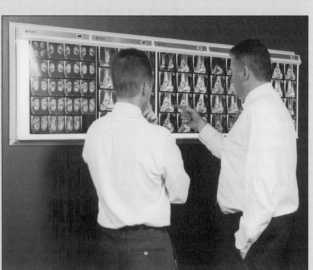

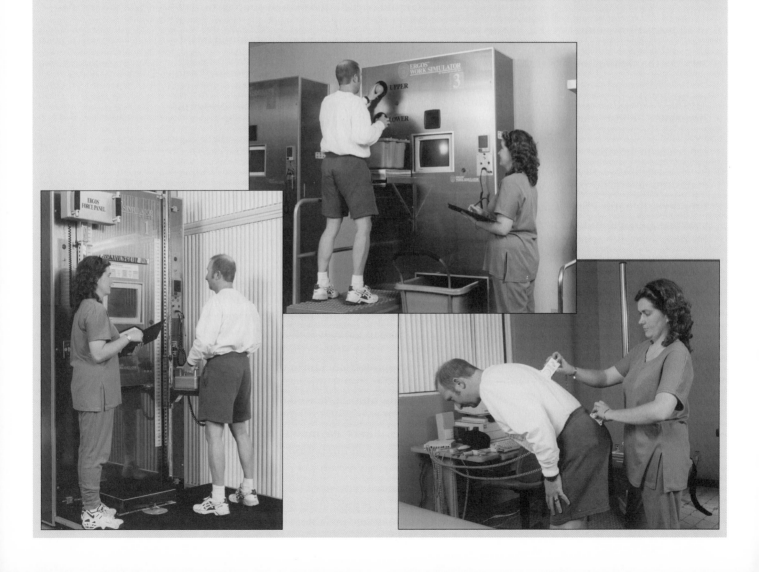

- 75% of workers had coverage for chiropractic services under their plans.

- 81–84% with conventional plans, PPOs and point-of-service plans had coverage.

- Only 44% of those with HMO plans had coverage.

A 1994 Group Health Association of America survey was consistent with the above in reporting that 46% of workers with HMO plans had chiropractic benefits.[41] That figure will be higher by now.

5. **Methods of Coverage.** How chiropractic services are covered obviously varies from policy to policy and from plan to plan. All of the following variations are found:

   a) *Health Services Account (HSA), Medical Savings Account (MSA) or flex plan:* The employee receives a set amount per annum for all health care services and can choose how much to spend on any of the various covered services including chiropractic. This method of coverage is gaining in popularity among employers and employees.

   b) *Group of Services:* A modification of the above. An employee gets a dollar amount for a group of non-medical service—e.g. all non-medical licensed services; all physical treatments (chiropractic, massage, physical therapy, acupuncture); chiropractic/vision services, etc. Coverage per visit may be total or part only with a patient copayment.

   c) *Full Chiropractic Services:* Coverage for full chiropractic services as a core benefit of the insurance plan on an equivalent basis to medical coverage. The precise extent of coverage for both chiropractic and medical services will depend upon the contract, and may or may not involve a co-payment by the patient. This type of coverage is the most desirable from the point of view of patients because it affords them equal access to the services of their choice.

   d) *Limited Chiropractic Services:* Coverage only for specified diagnostic services plus chiropractic manipulation.

   e) *Authorized Chiropractic Services:* Coverage only after prior authorization - e.g. by a nurse or medical gatekeeper (PCP) in an HMO. This is obviously the most restric-

Table 6 **Results of the RAND and American Chiropractic Association Studies**

Payment Source	RAND Study[1] (% of patients)	ACA Survey[2] (% of income)
Direct payments from patients (cash)	20.9	27.7
Private Insurance (Indemnity)	41.8	28.6
Auto insurance	9.8	14.5
Workers' Compensation	10.4	10.8
Medicare	7.3	8.4
Prepaid/Managed Care	3.7	8.6
Medicaid	1.5	1.2
Other	2.3	0.9

1 Source: Hurwitz EL, Coulter ID, Adams AH, Genovese BJ, Shekelle PG. Utilization of chiropractic services in the United States and Canada: 1985-1991. Am J Pub Health 88(5):771–6.

2 Source: Goertz C. Summary of 1995 annual statistical survey on chiropractic practice. J Am Chiro Assoc 1996;33(6):35–41

Table 7 **U.S. Employees with Insurance Coverage for Chiropractic Services in 1993**

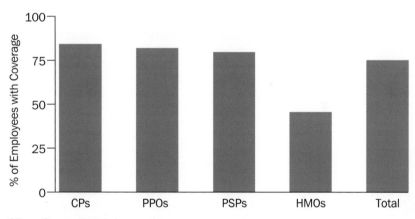

CPs = Conventional plans
PPOs = Preferred provider organizations or networks
PSPs = Point-of-service plans
HMOs = Health maintenance organizations
Total = Total employees with coverage

	Millions of Workers	Workers with Chiropractic Benefits	Workers without Chiropractic Benefits	Coverage Status Uncertain
Total	68.8	75%	19%	0.04
Among workers in:				
Conventional plans	33.7	84%	11%	
HMOs	15.1	44%	45%	
PPOs	13.8	83%	13%	
Point-of-service plans	6.2	81%	13%	

Source: Jensen G et al., citing the 1993 KPMG Peat Marwick/Wayne State University Survey of 1,953 Employers.[38]

tive form of coverage, with barriers to patient choice and access to services. It is often combined with other practices or incentives used to limit care.

For a fuller discussion of insurance coverage of chiropractic services in the U.S. see Jensen.[31]

References

1   Rosenberg v Cahill. 99 NJ 318, 492 A.2nd 371, 1985
2   Chapman-Smith DA. Legislative approaches to the regulation of the chiropractic profession. JCCA 1996;40:108–14.
3   Jackson R. Foreword. In Foreman SM, Croft CA. Whiplash injuries: The cervical acceleration/deceleration syndrome. Baltimore, Maryland: Williams and Wilkins, 1988.
4   Yochum TR, Rowe LJ. Essentials of skeletal radiology. Baltimore, Maryland: Williams and Wilkins, 1987.
5   Book Review. In NEJM 1996;334:1675.
6   Marchiori DM. Clinical imaging with skeletal, chest and abdomen pattern differentials. St. Louis, Missouri: Mosby, 1999.
7   Stude DE. Spinal rehabilitation. Stamford, Connecticut: Appleton & Lange. 1999.
8   Bergmann T, Peterson D, Lawrence D. Chiropractic technique: principles and procedures. New York: Churchill Livingstone, 1993.
9   Byfield D. Chiropractic manipulative skills. Oxford, England: Butterworth-Heinemann Ltd., 1996.
10 Bergmann TF, Davis PT. Mechanically assisted manual techniques: distraction procedures. St. Louis, Missouri: Mosby Yearbook Inc., 1998.
11 Hammer WI. Functional soft tissue examination and treatment by manual methods: new perspectives. 2nd edition. Gaithersburg, Maryland: Aspen. 1999.
12 Haldeman S, ed. Principles and practice of chiropractic. 2nd ed. Norwalk, Connecticut and San Mateo, California: Appleton and Lange, 1992.
13 Liebenson C, ed. Rehabilitation of the spine: a practitioner's manual. Baltimore, Maryland: Williams and Wilkins, 1996.
14 Murphy DR. Conservative management of cervical spine syndromes. New York: McGraw-Hill. 1999.
15 Lawrence DH, ed. Fundamentals of chiropractic diagnosis and management. Baltimore, Maryland: Williams & Wilkins. 1991.
16 Souza TA. Differential diagnosis for the chiropractor: protocols and algorithms. Gaithersburg, Maryland: Aspen, 1997
17 Cramer GD, Darby SA. Basic and Clinical anatomy of the spine, spinal cord and ANS. St. Louis, Missouri: Mosby Yearbook Inc, 1995.
18 Giles LGF, Singer KP, eds. Clinical anatomy and management of low-back pain. Oxford, England: Butterworth Heinemann, 1997.
19 Vernon H. Upper cervical syndrome: chiropractic diagnosis and treatment. Baltimore, Maryland: Williams & Wilkins, 1998.
20 Curl DD, ed. Chiropractic approach to head pain. Baltimore, Maryland: Williams & Wilkins, 1994.
21 Anrig C, Plaugher G. Pediatric Chiropractic. Baltimore, Maryland: Williams & Wilkins. 1997.
22 Souza TA, ed. Sports injuries of the shoulder: conservative management. New York: Churchill Livingstone, 1994.
23 Hyde TE, Gengenbach M, eds. Conservative Management of Sports Injuries. Baltimore, Maryland: Williams and Wilkins, 1997.
24 Kirkaldy-Willis WH, ed. Managing low-back pain. 3rd ed. New York: Churchill Livingstone, 1992.
25 Wall PD, Melzack RM. Textbook of pain. Orlando, Florida: W.B. Saunders, 1999.
26 Frymoyer JW, Ducker TB et al. The adult spine. Hagerstown, Maryland: Lippincott, Williams & Wilkins, 1996.
27 Hochschuler S, Reznik B. Treat your back without surgery: the best non-surgical alternatives to eliminating back and neck pain. Alameda, California: Hunter House Publishers. 1998.
28 Thompson CJ. Second report, Medicare Benefits Review Committee. Canberra, Australia: Commonwealth Government Printer, June 1986: Chapt. 10 (Chiropractic).
29 Complementary medicine: new approaches to good practice. Oxford, England: British Medical Association, Oxford University Press, 1993; 138.
30 Hurwitz EL, Coulter ID, Adams AH, Genovese BJ, Shekelle PG. Utilization of chiropractic services in the United States and Canada: 1985-1991. Am J Pub Health 1998;88(5):771–6.
31 Mierau DL, Cassidy JD, et al. Sacroiliac joint dysfunction and low back pain in school aged children. J Manip Physiol Ther 1984;7:81–4.
32 Leboeuf-Yde C, Ohm Kyvik L. At what age does low-back pain become a common problem? Spine 1998;23:228–34.
33 Triano J, Schultz AB. Loads transmitted during lumbosacral spinal manipulative therapy. Spine 1997;22:1955–64.
34 Thompson CJ. Second Report, Medicare Benefits Review Committee. Canberra, Australia: Commonwealth Government Printer, June 1986:Chapt. 10 (Chiropractic)
35 Hasselberg PD. Chiropractic in New Zealand, Report of A Commission of Inquiry. Wellington, New Zealand: Government Printer, 1979.
36 Commission on Alternative Medicine, Social Departementete, Legitimization for Vissa Kiropraktorer, Stockholm, SOU (English Summary) 1987:12-13–16.
37 Manga P, Angus D, et al. The effectiveness and cost-effectiveness of chiropractic management of low-back pain. Ottawa, Ontario: Pran Manga and Associates, University of Ottawa, 1993; 65–70.
38 Jensen G, Morrisey MA, et al. The new dominance of managed care: insurance trends in the 1990s. Health Affairs 1997;16:125–36.
39 Roy R. Personal Communication, June 2, 1997
40 Goertz C. Summary of 1995 annual statistical survey on chiropractic practice. J Amer Chiro Assoc 1996;33(6):35–41
41 Group Health Association of America. HMO Industry Profile. Washington DC: GHAA, 1994.

CHAPTER 4

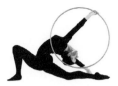

EDUCATION AND LICENSURE

A. Introduction

There is much misunderstanding of the extent and quality of chiropractic education. Recent focus groups held in Canada and the U.S. found that many members of the public thought that chiropractic education was about 2 years in duration, was greatly inferior to medical education and was basically chiropractors teaching chiropractors in unregulated private schools.

In fact in North America there is a minimum requirement of 6 years university-level training. All aspects of education must meet official accreditation standards, and a graduate must also complete state/provincial and national licensing board examinations before gaining the right to practice. Independent government and medical studies in the U.S.,[1,2] Sweden[3] and New Zealand[4] have concluded that chiropractic education is the equivalent of medical education in all of the basic sciences.

That is easy to prove in some cases. At the University of Odense in Denmark, for example, chiropractic and medical students take a basic sciences program in the same department for three years, with many shared subjects, lecturers and classes. They then divide into separate streams for clinical education.

Probably the most powerful concern medical doctors have about chiropractic, says Peter Curtis, MD, is "suspicion regarding the extent, depth and validity" of chiropractic education and "particularly the possibility of missing a serious disease." Dr. Curtis, from the Department of Family Practice at the University of North Carolina at Chapel Hill and writing in the *Journal of Family Practice*, reassures family physicians that "doctors of chiropractic are highly trained practitioners, qualified and licensed to diagnose disease entities and to refer patients when the treatment necessary is outside their scope of practice."[2] His conclusions were also those of the Swiss neurologist Dr. Jiri Dvorak after his investigation of U.S. chiropractic and medical schools in 1982[1] and the New Zealand Commission of Inquiry into Chiropractic after its visit to the U.S. and Canada in 1978.[4]

In January 1999 there were 31 chiropractic colleges worldwide recognized by the World Federation of Chiropractic and these are listed according to country at the end of this chapter in Appendix A. Other colleges are presently being established in various countries (e.g. Argentina, Chile, China, Italy, Malaysia, Mexico and the Philippines). All of these colleges adopt an international standard of education and require a minimum of four years full-time university-level education following entrance requirements.

Additionally, however, there are a number of chiropractic educational programs of lesser and inadequate standard in countries where the chiropractic profession is not regulated and the World Federation of Chiropractic (WFC) and the international chiropractic community have no authority. Examples are a second school in Brazil, and others in Taiwan, Germany and Japan, which has many such schools. In Sweden and the United Kingdom there are hybrid situations—schools recently recognized by the government but not as yet of international standard nor recognized by the WFC. (The U.K. has two such schools, the McTimoney and Oxford Colleges of Chiropractic, and three schools recognized by the WFC, the Anglo-European College of Chiropractic and schools at the Universities of Glamorgan and Surrey).

This chapter now reviews chiropractic education and licensure in the U.S. and Canada. Although most colleges are private institutions, whereas in other countries most colleges are in

Independent government and medical studies in the U.S., Sweden and New Zealand have concluded that chiropractic education is the equivalent of medical education in all of the basic sciences.

the publicly-funded university system, the content and standards of North American chiropractic education are representative of the international standard in recognized colleges.

B. Goals of Education

The basic goals of chiropractic education and licensure are to produce a primary-contact health care practitioner who is competent in the specific principles and practice of chiropractic and who is able to work both independently and in a health care team approach with other professionals as necessary. This means that there are three fundamentals:

... chiropractic colleges are not free to establish their own entrance requirements, curriculum, faculty and staff, governance, facilities, research and patient care. ... uniform minimum requirements are established through an official accreditation system.

1. A full grounding in anatomy, pathology and the other biological sciences on a similar basis to medical students.

2. The ability to perform a general or differential diagnosis, to assess health status and screen out patients requiring medical or other care and to perform a precise neuromusculoskeletal diagnosis as a basis for chiropractic care.

3. Education in the distinctive principles and skills of the chiropractic profession. (For details, see Chapter 5, "Principles and Goals of Chiropractic Care".)

C. Necessary Qualifications for the Right to Practice

All U.S. states and Canadian provinces have legislation regulating the practice of chiropractic. To practice a chiropractor requires a license from/registration with the licensing board, with the following preconditions:

1. Graduation from a duly accredited chiropractic college.

2. Completion of national board examinations.

3. Completion of state/provincial licensing board examinations. (For details see Section J, page 53.)

4. Satisfaction of various conditions common to licensed health professions, such as being of sound character, holding malpractice insurance and completing mandatory continuing education and/or practice review requirements.

Chiropractors are subject to discipline, including suspension or loss of license to practice, for professional misconduct. (For more on licensure see Section J.)

D. Accreditation

Although many chiropractic colleges are private institutions they are not free to establish their own entrance requirements, curriculum, faculty and staff, governance, facilities, research and patient care. In these and other areas, uniform minimum requirements are established through an official accreditation system.

In the U.S. the accrediting agency for the chiropractic profession is the Council on Chiropractic Education (CCE). It is based in Scottsdale, Arizona, and has been recognized by the U.S. Office of Education since 1974. In Canada it is the Canadian Council on Chiropractic Education (CCE Canada), which is formally affiliated with the CCE and has reciprocal standards.

All 16 U.S. chiropractic colleges, listed by region in Table 1, have accredited status with the CCE. (For full addresses, see Appendix A at the end of this chapter.) Additionally, 13 of them are accredited by non-chiropractic regional accrediting agencies such as the North Central Association of Schools and Colleges.

Canada has two schools of chiropractic. The Canadian Memorial Chiropractic College (CMCC) in Toronto is accredited and in the process of affiliation with York University. The School of Chiropractic at the University of Quebec, Trois Rivières Campus, founded in 1993, is a candidate for accreditation but is publicly funded and within the Quebec university system.

Accrediting agencies not only establish minimum standards but also assess institutional outcomes, effectiveness and continuing compliance with standards. The maximum period of accreditation is 7 years. Institutions provide annual reports, then, periodically, there are two more thorough review mechanisms:

1. Preparation and submission of a self-study of strengths, weaknesses and educational outcomes as they relate to CCE Standards.

2. Site visit and report to the CCE Commission on Accreditation by a CCE review team comprising educators and practitioners.

Table 1

West	Midwest	South	Northeast
Cleveland Chiropractic College Los Angeles Campus Los Angeles, CA *www.clevelandchiropractic.edu*	Cleveland Chiropractic College Kansas City Campus Kansas City, MO *www.clevelandchiropractic.edu*	Life College Marietta, GA *www.life.edu*	New York Chiropractic College Seneca Falls, NY *www.nycc.edu*
Life Chiropractic College West San Lorenzo, CA *www.life.edu*	Logan College of Chiropractic Chesterfield, MO *www.logan.edu*	Parker College of Chiropractic Dallas, TX *www.parkercc.edu*	University of Bridgeport College of Chiropractic Bridgeport, CT *www.bridgeport.edu/chiro*
Los Angeles College of Chiropractic Whittier, CA *www.lacc.edu*	National College of Chiropractic Lombard, IL *www.national.chiropractic.edu*	Sherman College of Straight Chiropractic Spartanburg, SC *www.shermansc.org*	
Palmer College of Chiropractic West San Jose, CA *www.palmer.edu*	Northwestern College of Chiropractic Bloomington, MN *www.nwchiro.edu*	Texas Chiropractic College Pasadena, TX *www.txchiro.edu*	
Western States Chiropractic College Portland, OR *www.wschiro.edu*	Palmer College of Chiropractic Davenport, IA *www.palmer.edu*	***For complete addresses and contact numbers, see Appendix A at the end of this chapter.***	

There are affiliated CCEs in Europe (the European Council on Chiropractic Education) and Australasia (the Australasian Council on Chiropractic and Osteopathic Education, governing schools in Australia and New Zealand). These and an *International Charter on Education* adopted by the World Federation of Chiropractic provide the basis for uniform minimum standards internationally. Despite this, however, the practice of chiropractic remains unregulated by law in a number of countries where lay persons can still practice as "chiropractors" without an accredited education.

E. Admission Requirements for Chiropractic Education

CCE requirements include a minimum of 2 years of undergraduate college education with a grade of C (a 2.5 grade point) or better in specified subjects—biology, general chemistry, organic chemistry, physics, psychology, English/communication and the humanities (CCE, 1995).

Entrance standards are also influenced by licensing board requirements. Currently six U.S. state boards require a bachelor's degree in addition to a doctor of chiropractic degree for licensure.

In fact, chiropractic colleges generally exceed CCE requirements. In the U.S., according to a study published in 1997:

1. The cumulative grade point average for all colleges was 2.90.

2. 42.2% of all applicants accepted had a bachelor's degree on entrance.[5]

In Canada, with only two colleges and greater competition for entrance, all successful candidates have at least three years of undergraduate study, over 80% have bachelor's degrees and the grade point average is 3.3.

F. Undergraduate Professional Program[6,7,8]

Length. This is a program of four academic years that is typically taught in either a year-round trimester program (see Table 2—all but the internship completed in 3 years) or a semester program (see Table 3—program content spread more evenly over 4 years). The minimum number of hours, as required by CCE for accreditation, is 4,200. In fact, hours at U.S. colleges range from 4,400 to 5,220 hours and average 4,822.

Figure 1 **Undergraduate Professional Program at Chiropractic Colleges**

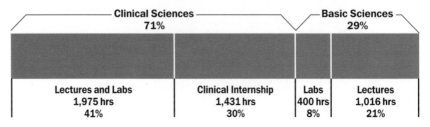

Clinical Sciences 71%		Basic Sciences 29%	
Lectures and Labs 1,975 hrs 41%	Clinical Internship 1,431 hrs 30%	Labs 400 hrs 8%	Lectures 1,016 hrs 21%

Table 2 **Subjects Taught in a Typical Trimester-based Chiropractic Program, by Year and Numbers of Contact Hours**

Year 1	Year 2	Year 3	Year 4
General anatomy (210)	Pharmacotoxicology (30)	Integrated chiropractic clinical application (90)	Clinical internship (450)
Functional anatomy and biomechanics (210)	Clinical microbiology (90)	Physiological therapeutics (30)	
Histology (90)	Pathology (135)	Chiropractic principles (75)	
Human biochem (105)	Chiropractic principles (60)	Practice management (75)	
Chiropractic principles (90)	Chiropractic procedures (300)	Imaging interpretation (90)	
Clinical chiropractic (60)	Physics and clinical imaging (90)	Radiological position and technique (30)	
Palpation (120)	Clinical orthopedics and neurology (180)	Differential diagnosis (90)	
Neuroscience (120)	Nutritional assessment (60)	Clinical application of manual procedures (60)	
Normal radiological anatomy (90)	Community health (60)	Clinical internship (390)	
Human physiology (135)	Physiological therapeutics (105)	Dermatology (15)	
Fundamentals of nutrition (60)	Clinical nutrition (60)	Clinical psychology (15)	
Introduction to physical examination skills (120)	Research methods (30)	Obstetrics/gynecology (15)	
Chiropractic procedures (105)	Practice management (30)	Pediatrics (15)	
	Imaging interpretation (75)	Geriatrics (15)	
	Differential diagnosis (90)	Clinical laboratory clerkship (15)	
	Clinical chiropractic applied (90)		
Total hours: 1,515	Total hours: 1,485	Total hours: 1,410	Total: 450
Total hours over four years: 4,860.			

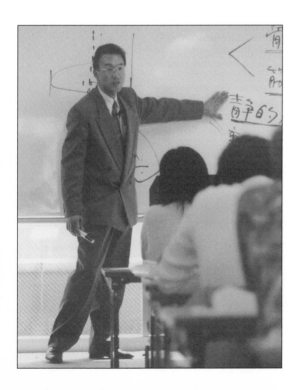

A lecture and clinical education at the RMIT University School of Chiropractic, Tokyo, Japan,

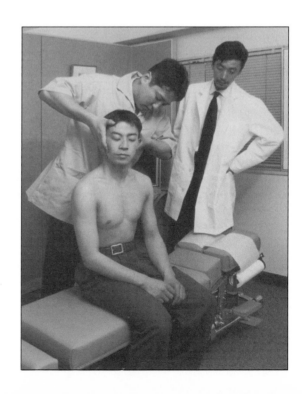

Table 3 **Sample Semester-based Curriculum at an Accredited Chiropractic College**

Division	First Year	Hrs	Second Year	Hrs	Third Year	Hrs	Fourth Year	Hrs
Biological Sciences	Human Anatomy Microscopic Anatomy Neuroanatomy Neuroscience (I) Biochemistry Physiology (I)	180 140 72 32 112 36	Pathology Lab Diagnosis (I) Microbiology & Infectious Diseases Neuroscience (II) Nutrition Immunology	174 40 100 87 58 13	Lab Diagnosis (II) Toxicology	32 13	Clinical Nutrition Community Health	26 39

Chiropractic Sciences	Chiropractic
	  Principles (I)
	Basic Body
	  Mechanics
	Chiropractic Skills (I)
		56
		
		96
		100
			Chiropractic
			  Principles (II)
			Chiropractic Skills (II)
			Spinal Mechanics
				58
				145
				42
					Chiropractic
					  Principles (III)
					Clinical Biomechanics
					Chiropractic Skills (III)
					Auxiliary Chiropractic
					  Therapy
					Introduction to Juris-
					  prudence & Prac-
					  tice Development
						42
						100
						145
						
						58
						
						16
							Integrated Chiro-
							  practic Practice
							Jurisprudence &
							  Practical
							  Develoment
								95
								
								46

Clinical Sciences	Normal Radio-
	  graphic Anatomy
	Radiation Biophysics
	  and Protection
		16
		
		44
			Intro. Diagnosis
			Intro. Bone Pathology
			Normal Roentgen.
			  Variants &
			  Roentgenometrics
				87
				48
				
				39
					Orthopedics &
					  Rheumatology
					Neurodiagnosis
					Differential
					  Diagnosis
					Diagnosis & Sympto-
					  matology
					Radiological
					  Technology
					Arthritis & Trauma
						92
						42
						
						32
						
						116
						
						39
						48
							Clinical Psychology
							Emergency Care
							Child Care
							Female Care
							Geriatrics
							Abdomen, Chest &
							  Special Radio-
							  graphic Procedures
								46
								52
								20
								29
								20
								
								40

Clinical Education	Observer (I)		Observer (II)		Observer (III)	406	Internship
							Auxiliary Chiropractic
							  Therapy Clerkship
							Clinical Lab Clerkship
							Clinical X-ray
							  Technology
							Clinical X-ray
							  Interpretation
							Chiropractic
							  Management
							Observer (IV)
								752
								
								33
								21
								
								21
								
								69
								
								31

Research					Applied Research
					  & Biometrics
						32	Research Investi-
							  gative Project	

TOTALS		912		978		1213		1390

Total hours over four years: 4,493

Basic Structure. The program is divided into:

1. *Basic Sciences.* These represent 1,416 hours on average, and 29% of the program. This involves lecture (1,016) and laboratory (400) hours. Laboratory hours in anatomy, for example, include human dissection.

2. *Clinical Sciences.* These represent an average of 3,406 hours and 71% of the program. They are divided into clinical education (average of 1,975 hours—including instruction in hands-on manual techniques for diagnosis and treatment) and a clinical clerkship (1,431 hours—patient management under supervision in outpatient clinics).

G.   Comparison with Medical Education

1. *Structure.* See Table 4 for a comparison of overall structure. The data used there comes from a recent study of all chiropractic and medical schools in the U.S., with detailed analysis of three representative pairs of schools, one each in California, Iowa and Texas.[7] Points of note include:

   - Chiropractic and medical schools have similar total student contact hours—4,822 (chiropractic) and 4,667 (medical).

   - Basic sciences represent 25–30% in each program. There is a similar amount of biochemistry, microbiology and pathology. Chiropractic students have significantly more anatomy and physiology, but many fewer hours in public health. Chiropractic and medical students use the same textbooks in these subjects.

   - Clinical science hours are also similar in total—3,406 (71%) and 3,467 (74%) respectively in chiropractic and medicine. However there is a major difference in how these are sub-divided. Chiropractic students divide clinical education between:

     chiropractic sciences or learning diagnostic and treatment methods (e.g. biomechanical diagnosis of the musculoskeletal system, manipulation and other manual treatment methods, and use of skeletal diagnostic x-ray and other imaging—1,975 hours or 41% of their total program); and

     clinical clerkship or supervised management of patients (1,431 hours or 30%).

   Medical undergraduate education has no equivalent of *chiropractic sciences.* All clinical science hours are spent in clinical clerkship (3,467 hours or 74% of the total program). Thus, on average, medical students receive over twice the number of hours of clinical experience.

   - In addition, medical students go on to residency training in hospitals and community-based practices. This raises the total number of hours of clinical experience for medical students to 6,413 hours.

   - These differences make sense. Chiropractic students are being prepared for a specialized primary contact or primary care role. As with similar professionals, such as dentists and optometrists, chiropractors need to acquire specialized treatment skills at undergraduate level but do not need the same depth of exposure to disease states as medical doctors.

2. *Emphasis.* In comparing the details of chiropractic and medical curricula there are other appropriate and expected differences. To name a few, with reference to the chiropractic program detailed in Table 3:

   - Subjects found in both the chiropractic and medical curricula are taught with a different emphasis. For example, first year study of anatomy in chiropractic emphasizes the musculoskeletal system (which represents 60% of the body but receives much less emphasis in medical education), the nervous system (neuroanatomy) and their interrelationship because these are of fundamental importance to chiropractic principles and scope of practice.

   - There are different areas of study. In chiropractic education there is little on pharmacology and surgery—merely an overview and introduction—because use of prescription drugs and surgery are not within the scope of practice of chiropractic. However these subjects are replaced with chiropractic sciences, subjects such as biomechanics and manual diagnostic and treatment methods for which there is little if anything comparable in medical education. For example:

a) Over the first 3 years there are 341 hours of biomechanics—general, spinal and clinical. (See Table 3, *Chiropractic Sciences*.)

b) Under Chiropractic Skills (see Table 3, *Chiropractic Sciences*) and Clinical Observation (see Table 3 *Clinical Education*) there are over 750 hours in the first 3 years providing groundwork in manual diagnostic and treatment methods. This lays the foundation for the clinical internship or clerkship in the fourth year.

c) Because the general practice of chiropractic involves the use of diagnostic x-ray, like dentistry but unlike medicine, there is thorough education in radiology. (See Table 3 *Clinical Sciences* and *Clinical Education*.)

As is explained by Karel Lewit, a neurologist self-trained in manipulation, disturbed mechanics or function in the musculoskeletal system is the single most common cause of pain syndromes for patients but has never formed part of the curriculum in medical education—either in undergraduate or postgraduate specialty education.[9] The professions of chiropractic and osteopathy have grown, Lewit concludes, largely because of this major gap in medical education and practice.

That gap is illustrated in a recent exercise in which orthopedic residents at the University of Pennsylvania Medical School were given and generally failed the competency exam in musculoskeletal medicine.[10]

H. Faculty

Quality of education depends not only upon the curriculum but also the competence of the faculty. Faculty qualifications and student-faculty ratios are also governed by CCE minimum standards. These require, for example, that basic sciences faculty must have at least a master's degree or doctorate in their discipline, and that clinical sciences faculty must have relevant academic and practical qualifications. Most colleges far exceed the minimum qualifications. At the Canadian Memorial Chiropractic College, the program for which is given in Table 3:

Table 4 **Comparisons of the Overall Curriculum Structure for Chiropractic and Medical Schools**

	Chiropractic Schools		Medical Schools	
	Mean	Percentage	Mean	Percentage
Basic Science Hours	1416	29%	1200	26%
Clinical Science Hours	3406	71%	3467	74%
Total Contact Hours	4822	100%	4667	100%
Sub-division of Clinical Science Hours				
Chiropractic Science Hours	1975	41%	0	0
Clerkship Hours	1431	30%	3467	74%
Total	3406	71%	3467	74%

Adapted from Coulter I, Adams A, et al. 1998.[6]

1. There are 115 faculty members, 53 full-time and 62 part-time, for a student population of 585.

2. Teaching the basic sciences are 13 PhDs (one also an MD, two also DCs) and 4 faculty members with MScs (one also a DC).

3. Doctors of chiropractic on the faculty who hold only the DC degree (29) or a DC and a bachelor degree (33) are teaching the chiropractic clinical sciences and/or supervising clinical education. Many of them also have chiropractic fellowships—postgraduate specialty qualifications.

I. Postgraduate Specialization

Postgraduate training is available in a variety of disciplines and specialties. This may be in full-time residency programs at chiropractic colleges (typically a minimum of 4,000 hours over two academic years—e.g. radiology) or part-time in non-residency programs offered by colleges and professional bodies (typically a minimum of 300 hours over three years—e.g. rehabilitation, sports chiropractic). Postgraduate degrees, fellowships and diplomates are available in:

Chiropractic Sciences
Diagnosis
Neurology
Nutrition
Occupational health
Orthopedics
Pediatrics
Radiology
Rehabilitation
Sports chiropractic
Thermography

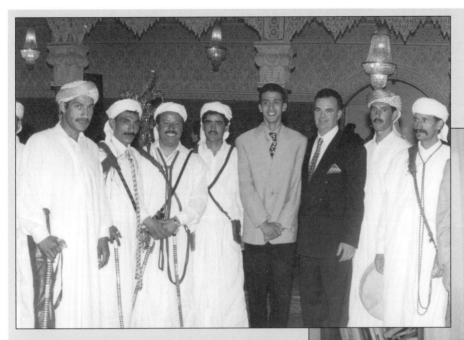

SPORTS CHIROPRACTIC

Chiropractors specializing in sports chiropractic treat average and élite athletes for three reasons—performance enhancement through better freedom of joint and muscle action, injury prevention, and management of injuries. Hicham El-Geurrouj of Morocco, world champion and record-holder in the 1500 meters and 1 mile (3:43.13), travels to competitions with his chiropractor, Dr. Jelloul Belhouari of Casablanca. Dr. Belhouari, now official chiropractor for the Moroccan track and field team and national soccer team, is pictured here with El-Geurrouj at a Royal reception in 1997, with Nezha Bidouane, 1997 world champion in the women's 400 meters, and at work at the 1998 World Cup in France.

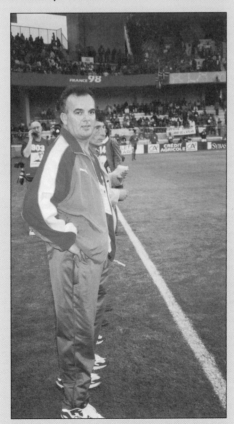

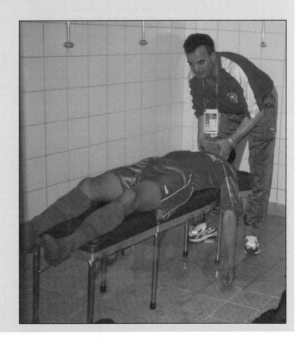

The single most developed postgraduate specialty in chiropractic is radiology, and in Chapter 3 there was mention of texts by chiropractic radiologists that have been reviewed by medical radiologists as state-of-the-art in skeletal radiology. Marchiori's text[11] combines chapters by chiropractic and medical radiologists (see pg. 33). The most rapidly developing specialties during the past 10 years, with the most students enrolled, are rehabilitation and sports chiropractic. The rehabilitation specialty draws upon active rehabilitation, methods developed in several disciplines, as illustrated in the text by Liebenson.[12]

J. Licensure

In North America and elsewhere where the practice of chiropractic is regulated by law, a graduate chiropractor must pass national and state/provincial licensing board examinations prior to receiving a license to practice.

In the United States:

1) Nearly 800 occupations are regulated by state licensing authorities.

2) For chiropractic there are state regulatory agencies with examining boards comprising DCs, lay persons, and/or MDs. A DC seeking a license to practice must pass the following board exams:

   - **Part I**—basic science in 6 areas (general anatomy, spinal anatomy, physiology, chemistry, pathology, microbiology and public health).

   - **Part II**—clinical science in 6 areas (general diagnosis, neuro-musculoskeletal diagnosis, X-ray, principles of chiropractic, chiropractic practice and associated clinical sciences).

   - **Part III**—clinical competency in 9 areas (case history, physical examination, neuromusculoskeletal examination, roentgenologic examination, clinical laboratory and special studies examination, diagnosis/clinical impression, chiropractic techniques, supportive techniques and case management).

3) It is not commonly known that prior to 1965, at a time when chiropractic examining boards had fewer resources, *chiropractors in most U.S. states took the same basic science board examinations as medical doctors.* Accordingly they were required to meet the same standard. Since that time chiropractic examinations have become separate while remaining at an equivalent standard with medicine.

4) The regulatory process for chiropractic education and practice has created two national organizations:

   a) **The Federation of Chiropractic Licensing Boards (FCLB).** (See page 28 for address.) The FCLB, established in 1933, seeks to unify standards and requirements of individual state boards and publishes their state licensure requirements annually. It is affiliated with, and has appointed members on:

   b) **The National Board of Chiropractic Examiners (NBCE).** (See page 28 for address.) The NBCE, established in 1963, has developed sophisticated examination systems that are now used nationally and internationally. Parts I, II and III described above were developed by the NBCE. Currently 46 states require or accept NBCE exams for licensure, others have requirements similar to, or modeled on, the NBCE exams.

. . . prior to 1965, chiropractors in most U.S. states took the same basic science board examinations as medical doctors. Since that time chiropractic examinations have become separate while remaining at an equivalent standard with medicine.

The author acknowledges that a valuable source for much information found in this chapter was Chiropractic Training, *by* **Coulter ID, Adams AH and Sandefur, R**, *Chapter 3 in* Chiropractic In The United States: Training, Practice and Research, *edited by* **Cherkin DC and Mootz RD**. *For the full reference to that book, see Reference 1 on page 8.*

References

1 Dvorak J. Manual medicine in the United States and Europe in the year 1982. Man Med 1983;3–9.
2 Curtis P, Bove G. Family physicians, chiropractors and back pain. J Fam Pract 1992;35(5):551–5.
3 Commission on Alternative Medicine, Social Departementete,'Legitimization for Vissa Kiropraktorer, Stockholm, SOU (English Summary) 1987:12-13-16.
4 Hasselberg PD. Chiropractic in New Zealand, Report of Commission of Inquiry. Wellington, New Zealand: Government Printer, 1979; 130–1,198.
5 Doxey TT, Phillips RB. Comparison of entrance requirements for health care professions, J Manip Physiol Ther 1997;20:86–91.
6 An evaluation of federal funding policies and programs and their relationship to the chiropractic profession. Arlington, Virginia: Foundation for Chiropractic Education and Research, Corporate Health Policies Group. 1991; 75–99.
7 Coulter I, Adams A, et al. A comparative study of chiropractic and medical education. Alt Ther in Health Med 1998;4:64–75.
8 McNamee P, ed. The chiropractic college directory, 1998. Los Angeles, California: KM Enterprises, 1997.
9 Lewit K. Manipulative therapy in rehabilitation of the locomotor system, 3rd ed. Oxford, England: Butterworth Heinemann, 1999. Chapter 10.
10 Freedman KB, Bernstein J. The adequacy of medical school education in musculoskeletal medicine. J Bone Joint Surg 1998;80-A:1421–7. (For further details on education required for the practice of manipulation see Chapter 7, Section B, page 100.)
11 Marchiori DM. Clinical imaging: with skeletal chest and abdomen pattern differentials. St Louis, Missouri: Mosby Yearbook, 1999.
12 Liebenson C, ed. Rehabilitation of the spine: a practitioner's manual. Baltimore, Maryland: Williams and Wilkins, 1996.

APPENDIX A

RECOGNIZED CHIROPRACTIC COLLEGES

AUSTRALIA

MacQuarie University Centre for Chiropractic
Suite 222, Building E7A, Summerhill
N.S.W. 2109, Australia
Tel: 61-2-9850-9380 *Fax*: 61-2-9850-9389
Email: chiro@mq.edu.au
Website: www.chiro.mq.edu.au
Principal: Rodney Bonello, DC, DO

RMIT University, School of Chiropractic
Plenty Road, Bundoora
Victoria 3083, Australia
Tel: 61-3-9468-2440 *Fax*: 61-3-9467-2794
Email: A.Kleynhans@rmit.edu.au
Website: www.rmit.edu.au
Head of Department: Andries Kleynhans, DC
Head of School: Max Walsh, DC

BRAZIL

Feevale Central University
(Centro Universitario Feevale)
Rua Emillo Hauschild, 70-Villa Nova
Caixa postal 2121, Novo Hamburgo
RS-CEP 93525.180, Brazil
Tel: 55-51-594-2122 *Fax*: 55-51-594-7977
Website: www.feevale.tche.br
Administrator: Prof. Angela Kolberg

CANADA

Canadian Memorial Chiropractic College
1900 Bayview Avenue, Toronto
Ontario M4G 3E6 Canada
Tel: 1-416-482-2340 *Fax*: 1-416-482-9745
Email: jmoss@cmcc.ca
Website: www.cmcc.ca
President: Jean Moss, DC, MBA

**Université du Québec à Trois-Rivières—
   School of Chiropractic**
P.O. Box 500, 3351 Des Forges Boulevard
Trois-Rivières, Quebec G9A 5H7 Canada
Tel: 1-819-376-5186 *Fax*: 1-819-376-5204
Email: pierre_b_boucher@uqtr.uquebec.ca
Website: www: uqtr.uqebec.ca
Program Director: Pierre Boucher, DC, PhD

DENMARK

**University of Southern Denmark (Odense)
Faculty of Health Sciences**
Campusvej 55, DK-5230 Odense, Denmark
Tel: 45-66-158 600 *Fax*: 45-66-158 186
Email: n.nilsson@imbmed.ou.dk
Director of Chiropractic Studies: Niels Grunnet-Nilsson, DC MD PhD

FRANCE
Franco-European Chiropractic Institute
(Institut Franco-Européen de Chiropratique)
24 av. Paul Vaillant-Couturier
94200 Ivry-Sur-Seine, France
Tel: 33-1-45-15-8910 *Fax*: 33-1-45-15-8911
Email: ifec@chiropratique.org
Website: www.ifec.net
Director: M. Charles Martin
Academic Dean: Christophe Cordier, DC

JAPAN
RMIT University Chiropractic Unit—Japan
Shinbashi SD Building 4F
6-12-7 Shinbashi, Minato-ku
Tokyo 105, Japan
Tel: 81-3-3437-6907 *Fax*: 81-3-5401-0956
Head: Hiroaki Takeyachi, DC, MD

KOREA
Hanseo University: RMIT Chiropractic Division
136-220 Jaegi-2 Dong Dongdaemoon-Ku
Seoul, Korea
Tel: 82-2-924-8723 *Fax*: 82-2-924-9370
Email: chiropia@hotmail.com
Head: Associate Professor Hong Mo Yang

NEW ZEALAND
NZCA School of Chiropractic
P.O. Box 7144, Wellesley Street
Auckland 1, New Zealand
Tel: 64-9-373-4343 *Fax*: 64-9-373-5973
Head of School: Ralph Boone, DC, PhD

SOUTH AFRICA
Technikon Natal
Nattechnikon 6-20187
953 Durban 4000, South Africa
Tel: 27-31-224153 *Fax*: 27-31-223632
Email: gtill@umfolozi.ntech.ac.za
Head, Department of Chiropractic: A. Glynn Till, DC

Technikon Witwatersrand
P.O. Box 17011, Doorntontein 2028
Johannesburg, South Africa
Tel: 27-40-62911 *Fax*: 27-40-20475
Head of Department: Harold Humphries, DC

UNITED KINGDOM
Anglo-European College of Chiropractic
13-15 Parkwood Road
Bournemouth BH5 2DF, U.K.
Tel: 44-1202-436-275, *Fax*: 44-1202-436-312
Email: principal@aecc-chiropractic.ac.uk
Website: www.aecc_chiropractic.ac.uk
Principal: Gabriel Donleavy, PhD

University of Glamorgan,
School of Applied Sciences
Pontypridd, Wales CF37 1DL, U.K.
Tel: 44-1443-488-2294 *Fax*: 44-1443-482-2285
Principal: Susan King, DC, DHSM, MBS

University of Surrey, European Institute of Health
and Medical Sciences
Stirling House Campus, Stirling Road,
Surrey Research Park, Guildford, Surrey GU2 5RF, U.K.
Tel: 44-1483-302-239 *Fax*: 44-1483-259-748
Email: j.morley@surrey.ac.uk
Principal: Joseph Morley, DC

USA
Cleveland Chiropractic College,
Kansas City Campus
6401 N. Rockhill Road
Kansas City, Missouri 64131, USA
Tel: 1-816-333-8230 *Fax*: 1-816-361-0272
Website: www.clevelandchiropractic.edu
President: Carl S. Cleveland III, DC

Cleveland Chiropractic College,
Los Angeles Campus
590 North Vermont Avenue
Los Angeles, California 90004, USA
Tel: 1-213-660-6166 *Fax*: 1-213-660-5387
Website: www.clevelandchiropractic.edu
President: Carl Cleveland III, DC

Life University
1269 Barclay Circle, Marietta
Georgia 30060, USA
Tel: 1-770-424-0554 *Fax*: 1-770-429-4819
Email: admissions@life.edu
Website: www.life.edu
President: Sid E. Williams, DC

Life Chiropractic College-West
2005 Via Barrett, P. O. Box 367
San Lorenzo, California 94580, USA
Tel: 1-510-276-9013 *Fax*: 1-510-276-6798
Email: info@lifewest.edu
Website: www.lifewest.edu
President: Gerard W. Clum, DC

Logan College of Chiropractic
1851 Schoettler Road, Box 1065
Chesterfield, Missouri 63006-1065, USA
Tel: 1-314-227-2100 *Fax*: 1-314-207-2420
Email: loganadm@logan.edu
Website: www.logan.edu
President: George A. Goodman, DC

Los Angeles College of Chiropractic
16200 E. Amber Valley Drive, P.O. Box 1166
Whittier, California 90609, USA
Tel: 1-562-947-8755 *Fax*: 1-562-947-5724
Email: lacc@deltanet.com
Website: www.lacc.edu
President: Reed Phillips, DC, PhD

National College of Chiropractic
200 E. Roosevelt Road
Lombard, Illinois 60148, USA
Tel: 1-630-629-2000 *Fax*: 1-630-889-6554
Email: homepage@nationalchiropractic.edu
Website: www.national.chiropractic.edu
President: James F. Winterstein, DC

New York Chiropractic College
2360 State Route 89, P.O. Box 800
Seneca Falls, New York 13148-0800, USA
Tel: 1-315-568-3000 *Fax*: 1-315-568-3015
Website: www.nycc.edu
President: Kenneth Padgett, DC

Northwestern Health Sciences University
2501 West 84th Street
Bloomington, Minnesota 55431, USA
Tel: 1-612-888-4777 *Fax*: 1-612-888-6713
Email: admit@nwchiro.edu
Website: www.nwchiro.edu
President: John Allenburg, DC

Palmer College of Chiropractic
1000 Brady Street
Davenport, Iowa, 52803, USA
Tel: 1-319-884-5000 *Fax*: 1-319-326-9897
Email: pcadmit@palmer.edu
Website: www.palmer.edu
President: Guy Riekeman DC

Palmer College of Chiropractic-West
90 East Tasmin Drive
San Jose, California 95134, USA
Tel: 1-408-944-6000 *Fax*: 1-408-944-6051
Website: www.palmer.edu
President: Peter Martin, DC

Parker College of Chiropractic
2500 Walnut Hill Lane
Dallas, Texas 75229-5668 USA
Tel: 1-972-438-6932 *Fax*: 1-972-357-3107
Website: www.parkercc.edu
President: Fabrizio Mancini, DC

Sherman College of Straight Chiropractic
P.O. Box 1452
Spartanburg, South Carolina 29304, USA
Tel: 1-864-578-8770 *Fax*: 1-864-599-7145
Email: admissions@shermansc.org
Website: www.shermansc.org
President: David B. Koch, DC

Texas Chiropractic College
5912 Spencer Highway
Pasadena, Texas 77505, USA
Tel: 1-281-487-1170 *Fax*: 1-281-487-4168
Website: *www.txchiro.edu*
President: Shelby Elliott, DC

**University of Bridgeport,
College of Chiropractic**
75 Linden Avenue
Bridgeport, Connecticut 06601, USA
Tel: 1-203-576-4279 *Fax*: 1-203-576-4351
Website: www.bridgeport.edu/chiro
Dean: Frank Zolli, DC, EdD.

Western States Chiropractic College
2900 N.E. 132nd Avenue
Portland, Oregon 97230, USA
Tel: 1-503-256-3180 *Fax*: 1-503-251-5723
Email: admissions@wschiro.edu
Website: www.wschiro.edu
President: William H. Dallas, DC

CHAPTER 5

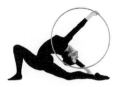

PRINCIPLES AND GOALS OF CHIROPRACTIC CARE

A. Introduction and Definition

The medical profession and most members of the public usually identify chiropractors and chiropractic practice with joint manipulation for the relief of back pain and other musculoskeletal pain. Two recent studies from North America confirm that this is an accurate reflection of chiropractic practice.[1,2] Approximately 2 of every 3 patients have back pain, and 9 of 10 have one or more of back pain, neck pain, headache or pain in the extremities.

However chiropractic principles and practice are much more comprehensive than pain management. Patients seeing a chiropractor for musculoskeletal pain commonly experience other health benefits, such as relief from dysmenorrhea or chronic constipation, and medical doctors now understand that there may often be an important inter-relationship between dysfunction in the spine and locomotor system and dysfunction in other systems such as the circulatory, digestive and respiratory systems.[3]

This concept is discussed further in this chapter (see *Somatovisceral Effects*. page 62) and Chapter 6, "Scope of Practice."

The definition and paradigm of chiropractic practice, and the role of chiropractic in the health care system, have recently been described by two representative authorities in the profession.

1. The Association of Chiropractic Colleges (ACC): The ACC, which represents all 18 chiropractic colleges in North America, released a unanimous Position Paper in 1996 signed by the presidents of all colleges, with the intent of establishing a common position on the essentials of chiropractic education and practice. The ACC's chiropractic paradigm appears in Figure 1. Its definition of chiropractic is:

"*Chiropractic* is a health care discipline that emphasizes the inherent recuperative power of the body to heal itself without the use of drugs or surgery. The *practice of chiropractic* focuses on the relationship between structure (primarily the spine) and function (as coordinated by the nervous system) and how that relationship affects the preservation and restoration of health. In addition, doctors of chiropractic recognize the value and responsibility of working in cooperation

Figure 1 **The ACC Chiropractic Paradigm**

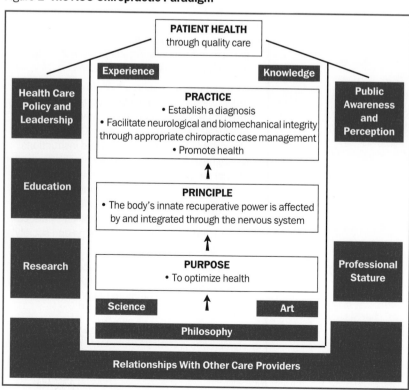

with other health care practitioners when in the best interest of the patient."

One significant element of this definition is the exclusion of drugs from chiropractic

practice. This is different from osteopathy in North America, which began as a drugless profession but changed in the 1960s. Many members of the medical profession have felt that chiropractic would pursue the use of prescription drugs. For reasons of principle, referred to in the above definition, and

Figure 2

The chiropractor in the primary health care system is a first-contact gate-keeper for neuro-musculoskeletal conditions.

Resolved, that the House of Delegates adopt the following as the American Chiropractic Association statement of policy on the Role of Chiropractic in Primary Health Care:

THE ROLE OF CHIROPRACTIC IN THE EVOLVING HEALTH CARE SYSTEM

The role of chiropractic in primary health care is characterized by direct access, longitudinal, integrated, conservative ambulatory care of patients' health care needs, emphasizing neuromusculoskeletal conditions, health promotion, and patient-centered diagnosis and management. The chiropractor in the primary health care system is a first-contact gate-keeper for neuromusculoskeletal conditions.

The principles outlined below are intended to better serve the health needs of the public. They also provide policy makers, other health care professionals and the public with a clear understanding of chiropractic. These principles are also intended to provide a focal point to which members of the profession can gravitate and will allow the profession to pursue its legitimate aspirations for growth and development.

- Chiropractors are first-contact physicians who possess the diagnostic skills to differentiate health conditions that are amenable to their management from those conditions that require referral or co-management.

- Chiropractors provide conservative management of neuromusculoskeletal disorders and related functional manifestations including, but not limited to, back pain, neck pain and headaches.

- Chiropractors are expert providers of spinal and other therapeutic manipulation/adjustments. They also utilize a variety of manual, mechanical and electrical therapeutic modalities. Chiropractors also provide patient evaluation and instructions regarding disease prevention and health promotion through proper nutrition, exercise and lifestyle modification among others. The range of diagnostic and therapeutic services offered by chiropractic is dynamic and will be modified by education, research, technological change and society's evolving health care needs.

- Chiropractic diagnostic and therapeutic goals should be achieved as safely, quickly and economically as possible to promote patient health and independence.

- Optimal patient care can best be achieved when chiropractic is vertically integrated within the health care system. Interdisciplinary collaboration is essential to this purpose.

- The diagnostic and therapeutic guidelines adopted by the profession should be evidence-based. In health care, the absence or ambiguity of scientific evidence requires using sound clinical judgement in place of hard data.

- Chiropractors offer accessible and appropriate care to all population groups.

- Chiropractic recognizes the multi-faceted aspects of health, disease, etiology and related patient care.

Glossary of Terms

Adjustment – Any chiropractic therapeutic procedure that utilizes controlled force, leverage, direction, amplitude and velocity which is directed at specific joints or anatomical regions.

Chiropractors commonly use such procedures to influence joint and neurophysiological function.

Conservative – Designed to preserve health, restore function, and repair structures by non-radical methods. In chiropractic, also implies the use of only drugless and nonsurgical methods.

Direct Access – Accessibility to services with one initial contact to a health care source.

Also implies that services are attainable within a reasonable time frame, that the services are affordable to those in the community and that the services are available to all who seek them.

First Contact – The point of entry into the health care system for the patient seeking care.

Also denotes that this point of entry is easily accessible to the patient, that it possesses services that can be used to address the patient's care needs, and that the patient can use these services for each new problem or recurrence of a problem that prompts the person to seek health care.

Gatekeeper – An individual who is the initial point of contact for the patient within a health care delivery facility. Also denotes one who is assigned responsibility for the initial assessment of the patient's needs, for treating or referring the patient as appropriate, for being accessible to the patient with a minimum of delay, and for being responsive to the urgency of the patient's needs.

Health promotion – An array of programs and services designed to enhance satisfaction and well-being.

continued on next page

Integrated – Organized into an inter-disciplinary facility or inter-disciplinary network of collaborating facilities that provides patient access to the type of provider and the level of services that the person requires with a minimum of delay. Also implies coordination of services necessary for problem recognition and appropriate management, maintenance of an accurate medical record and efficient use of resources.

Longitudinal – Able to provide for continuity of case management, including initial triage, treatment and coordination of specialty services, over the time course of necessary care to resolution or maximum therapeutic benefit. Presupposes patient accessibility to a health care source and the use of that source by the patient as the need arises.

Manipulation – A manual procedure that involves a directed thrust to move a joint past the physiological range of motion, without exceeding the anatomical limit.

Manipulable Subluxation – A subluxation in which altered alignment, movement and/or function can be improved by manual thrust procedures.

Motion Segment – A functional unit made up of the two adjacent articulation surfaces and the connecting tissues binding them to each other.

Neuromusculoskeletal – Function of the musculoskeletal system is integrated with neurological function and expressed by biological regulatory mechanisms.

Patient-Centered – An orientation to patient care that recognizes the many antecedents and cofactors in the disease and healing process, such as lifestyle, environment and genetics, and seeks to address those factors as an integral part of the patient's care.

Spinal Motion Segment – Two adjacent vertebrae and the connecting tissues binding them to each other.

Subluxation – A motion segment, in which alignment, movement integrity and/or physiological function are altered although contact between joint surfaces remains intact.

Subluxation Complex – A theoretical model of motion segment dysfunction (subluxation) which incorporates the complex interaction of pathological changes in nerve, muscle, ligamentous, vascular and connective tissues.

Subluxation Syndrome – An aggregate of signs and symptoms that relate to pathophysiology or dysfunction of spinal and pelvic motion segments or to peripheral joints.

Triage – To determine priority of need and proper placement of treatment.

Vertical integration – A system that provides for primary care, specialty care or hospitalization, as necessary, through interdisciplinary and specialty collaboration.

respect for the medical profession's scope of practice, it has not.

Another element of the ACC definition and paradigm, seen in the foundation of Figure 1, is recognition that chiropractors are part of an interdisciplinary health care system and have a responsibility to understand and work in collaboration with other health care practitioners.

2. *The American Chiropractic Association (ACA).* In 1994 the ACA adopted policy to "provide policy makers, other health care professionals and the public with a clear understanding of chiropractic" and "(its) role in the evolving health care system." The text of that policy appears in Figure 2. Technical terms are defined by the ACA in the Glossary of Terms. Again, as with the ACC, there is emphasis on drugless care and integration with other health care practitioners.

The rest of this chapter discusses key chiropractic principles in slightly greater depth

B. Essential Principles

Doctors of chiropractic often refer to "the philosophy, art and science of chiropractic" and in doing so are quoting the profession's founder, D.D. Palmer. The word *philosophy* is used with the meaning of essential guiding principles. These, as seen in the ACC Position Paper, have always been and remain:

1. **Holism**. This is a broadly accepted principle, reflected in the World Health Organization's definition of health as: "Health is a state of complete physical, mental, and social well-being and not merely the absence of disease or infirmity." The purpose of chiropractic care is not merely to relieve a symptom or address a cause of that symptom, important as these things may be to the patient, but to provide holistic care. It is to treat the whole person or, as the ACC paradigm says "to optimize health."

Therefore chiropractors use a variety of conservative (non-invasive, as opposed to drugs and surgery) methods of management including manual care, nutrition, exercises, advice on lifestyle and posture and patient counseling and motivation. Patients report high satisfaction rates—for back pain, three times the satisfaction rate for medical care[2] —partly because they now understand their problems and how to prevent future pain and disability in the context of their whole lives.

2. **Homeostasis.** Once more this is a basic and broadly accepted principle. It is that the body has its own inherent healing power and ability to resist disease. Its tendency is to return to normal health. The founding generation of chiropractors called this the "Innate" or "the power within." In the words of the ACC paradigm "the body's innate recuperative power is affected by and integrated through the nervous system."

. . . the body's innate recuperative power is affected by and integrated through the nervous system.

3. **The Primary Regulatory Role of the Nervous System**. The chiropractic profession places emphasis on the role of the nervous system in regulating function in all other systems of the body, and therefore in integrating homeostasis and general health. For teaching purposes the nervous system, which is one integrated system, is divided into three components:

    1. The central nervous system (CNS)—comprising the brain and spinal cord.

    2. The peripheral nervous system (PNS)—the nerves leading out from the spinal cord to the bones, joints, ligaments, muscles and skin of the soma or musculoskeletal system, and those bringing back to the CNS messages of pressure, position, balance and pain.

    3. The autonomic nervous system (ANS)—the nerves that regulate function of the internal or visceral organs (e.g. heart, liver, gastrointestinal system, sweat glands, etc.)

At each level in the spine there are combined or common processing centers in the spinal cord for the PNS (fed into by the spinal nerves at that vertebral level) and the ANS (fed into by autonomic nerves servicing other body organs and functions).

From their earliest clinical experiences, watching the various and often surprising ways in which patients respond to spinal manipulation, chiropractors have postulated that mechanical dysfunction in the musculoskeletal system, such as reduced range of motion and stiff joints or shortened or tense muscles, may disturb the normal regulatory function of all three branches of the nervous system—through these common spinal processing centers.

One possible mechanism for this, called central sensitization, is a continuing overexcited barrage of reflex responses into the processing systems in the CNS. Sophisticated animal experiments in recent years have shown that mechanical stimulation of spinal nerves not only causes reflex effects throughout the nervous system but also alters visceral function such as heart rate and adrenal activity.[3,4]

Accordingly, the goals of chiropractic joint adjustment or manipulation are not only to correct musculoskeletal dysfunction, improving range of motion and reducing pain, but also to restore normal function in the nervous system. This, chiropractors postulate, will improve homeostasis and thus affect body functions generally, improving resistance to disease and producing a feeling of well being. Much of this is yet to be proven convincingly, but it is consistent with modern neurophysiology and explains clinical results in chiropractic practice, such as the case below (see paragraph 6).

Finally, chiropractors have always acknowledged that spinal manipulation also influences other controlling systems, such as the circulatory and lymphatic systems. This was part of Palmer's original writings. However main emphasis has been placed on the nervous system. One reason for this will have been the early prosecutions of chiropractors for practicing osteopathy without a license. Osteopathy claimed that manipulation worked via the circulatory system, and part of the standard defence for chiropractors accused of practicing osteopathy early in the century was that they were working on the nervous system alone—and therefore practicing chiropractic.

4. **Subluxation.** This is the name chiropractors gave to the spinal joint lesion or dysfunction that they correct by manipulation or adjustment. It has been controversial with the medical profession because of a conflicting medical definition, but is today used by medical doctors who understand and use manipulation.[5,6] Medical critics have asked

how there can be a subluxation if it cannot be seen on x-ray. The answer is that the chiropractic subluxation is essentially a functional entity, not structural, and is therefore no more visible on static x-ray than a limp or headache or any other functional problem. Its components are:

1. Abnormal function/range of motion in a spinal joint

2. Neurological and/or vascular involvement

3. Often, but not necessarily, some structural displacement

A modern consensus definition, and the one adopted by the ACA (see Figure 2), is: "A motion segment in which alignment, movement integrity, and/or physiologic function are altered, although contact between the joint surfaces remains intact."[7]

The concept is not unique to chiropractic. Its equivalents are the "osteopathic lesion" and the "segmental blockage" of the European manual medicine school.

In medicine a joint subluxation is a clear orthopedic and structural lesion, something less than a full dislocation, always visible on x-ray. Because of this fertile ground for confusion, many chiropractors today who are working closely with medical doctors prefer the term "joint dysfunction." There is some irony in this because, in the eighteenth and nineteenth centuries, medical authors used the term subluxation in the chiropractic sense.[8]

Dysfunction in the musculoskeletal system may, of course, be in many tissues—muscles, connective tissue, fascia, ligaments. Subluxation or joint dysfunction has been given emphasis because of its central importance in chiropractic principle and practice.

5. **The Neuromusculoskeletal System (NMS System)**. Chiropractors signify the close relationship between the musculoskeletal tissues of the body and the nervous system by referring to the *neuromusculoskeletal system*. In treating this system they have two roles:

1. *Orthopedic*. This is understanding and addressing the mechanical function of the muscles and joints. Moving this joint

or releasing that muscle can free a tag of connective tissue caught in a joint and reduce pain. Better function in an arthritic joint can prevent wear and pain. In this role a chiropractor can be compared with the car mechanic, tuning the motor or aligning the front wheels.

2. *Neurologic*. Manipulating a joint also produces various reflex effects throughout the nervous system, and may have wider effects on symptoms and health. In this role a chiropractor is more like an

Chiropractors signify the close relationship between the musculoskeletal tissues of the body and the nervous system by referring to the neuromusculoskeletal system.

electrical engineer or telecommunications specialist.

Here is an example of a chiropractic approach to diagnosis and management based on the NMS system. Assume there is a patient with chronic headaches. He has no other disease or condition causing these headaches—in medical terms they are benign. However they are frequently incapacitating. Medical examination would look for a cause in the head (intracranial) and also consider lifestyle and psychological factors. Symptoms are likely to be managed with medication.

Chiropractic examination would also involve an assessment of the whole NMS system. In some patients the fundamental cause of the headaches may be a short leg, leading to imbalance of the pelvis at the base of the spine and compensations in the low-back and the neck or cervical spine. The immediate cause of the headaches is tension in the upper cervical spine, expressed as headache through tension on the pain-sensitive dura surrounding the spinal cord at the base of the skull.

For such patients treatment may be a foot orthotic or shoe lift for the short leg to balance the pelvis, and manipulation of the low-back. This may automatically resolve the compensating dysfunction in the cervical spine and the tension at that level causing the headaches. There may be need for

This promotional poster from the British Chiropractic Association (BCA) illustrates that, despite the potential benefits of chiropractic treatment for somatovisceral disorders such as Mrs. M's high blood pressure as discussed on the opposite page, the chiropractic profession's primary focus in daily practice is the management of musculoskeletal disorders. These are the type of disorders described on the poster. They represent 95% of chiropractic practice (see page 70) and are the conditions for which there is best scientific evidence of the effectiveness of chiropractic treatment. The BCA poster also illustrates the difference between European and North American sensibilities in the field of promotion.

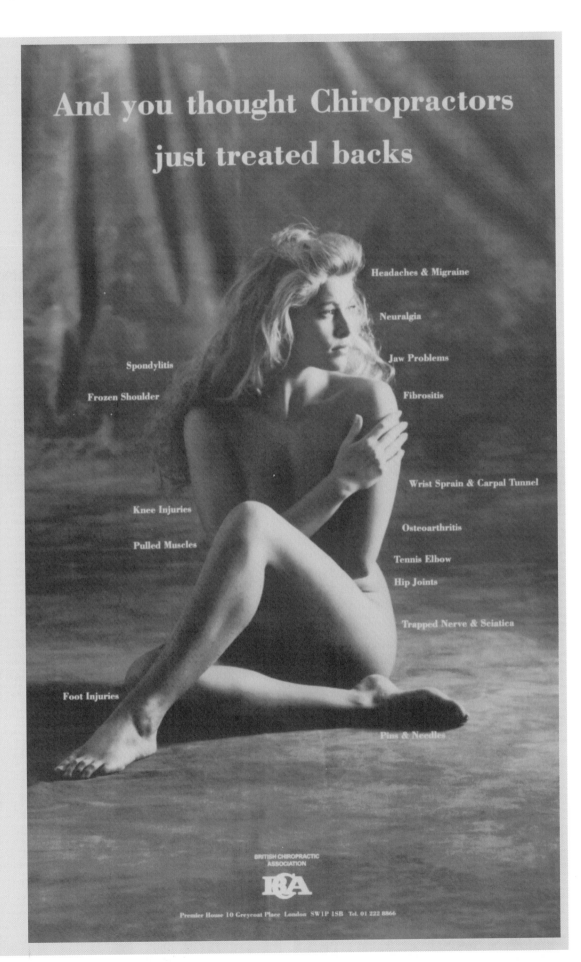

some joint and other soft-tissue mobilization or manipulation in the cervical spine.

6. **Somatovisceral Effects**. In the above example the one effect of treatment discussed so far, relief from headaches, is within the NMS system. But a further principle of chiropractic is that manual treatments of the NMS system or body framework (the soma) may influence the function of the internal body systems and organs (the viscera). This is because reflex effects in the nervous system include effects in the autonomic branch of the nervous system (ANS) which regulates visceral function. There is a large amount of new literature in this area, summarized in a recent text by Sato, Sato and Schmidt.[9] However this is a relatively small area of clinical practice, and there are presently fewer clinical trials than in the fields of musculoskeletal pain and headache.

Here is a case example, chosen because it was investigated by a judicial inquiry, was tested by medical cross-examination of the patient and independent findings were made and reported. Mrs. M consulted a chiropractor for neck pain and headache after whiplash injury. A course of chiropractic manipulation was successful.

In giving her history Mrs. M had told her chiropractor that she had been taking daily medication for 15 years for moderate hypertension and a related water retention problem, for which she remained under regular medical care. He had suggested that in response to his treatment the hypertension and edema might improve, with less need for continuing medication. As Mrs. M said at the hearing, she was sceptical of this. In fact, to the surprise of both her and her family physician, her blood pressure became normal and her anti-hypertensive medication was stopped, and her edema was greatly reduced requiring diuretic tablets once or twice a week rather than daily as previously.

The Commission recognized that no firm conclusions could be drawn in the circumstances. It was left with "facts and probabilities." Could chiropractic manipulation, like the anti-hypertensive medication, affect transmission in the post-ganglionic adrenergic nerves in the autonomic nervous system and produce a clinical result? The Commission concluded that "the treatment did have the effect both of relieving her hypertension and reducing her dependency on medication."[10]

For reference to more research in the area of somatovisceral effects see Chapter 6, Section C, pages 76–88.

C. Goals of Chiropractic Practice

The goals of chiropractic practice are seen in the above discussion and case examples. In summary they are:

1. To meet the patient's immediate needs, often the relief of pain.

2. To address the cause of the symptoms by restoring normal ranges of movement and function to the joints, muscles and other structures of the musculoskeletal or locomotor system.

3. By restoring function to the musculoskeletal system, and especially the joints of the spine, to allow the nervous system to function without interference and better regulate the various body systems and general health.

It is because of this linkage between the musculoskeletal system and the nervous system that chiropractors talk of the neuromusculoskeletal system and neuromusculoskeletal disorders.

If you understand these three goals of chiropractic health care, and that a chiropractor is concerned with more than relief of pain and other symptoms, you will understand why:

- When a patient is consulting a chiropractor for back pain or headache the chiropractor, adopting his/her professional viewpoint, is not treating back pain or headache but subluxation, joint dysfunction, trigger points or muscle imbalance.

- Chiropractors will treat some patients with asthma or hypertension or menstrual cramps or even ulcers—but say they are not treating those conditions. The basis for their care is mechanical dysfunction in the neuromusculoskeletal system. Clinical experience and research confirm that such dysfunction can contribute to or mimic many disorders that appear to be unconnected to the spine and the neuromusculoskeletal system as a whole.

- Chiropractors encourage periodic spinal examinations and preventive or wellness care. Their professional goal is normal function of the neuromusculoskeletal system for the prevention of pain and ill health. Some patients will choose this level of preventive care, others will not, in the same way that patients choose their level of preventive dental and medical care and their level of concern about a healthy lifestyle, good nutrition and exercise.

References

1   Position Paper. Association of Chiropractic Colleges. 1996.

2   Cherkin DC, MacCormack FA. Patient evaluation of low-back pain care from family physicians and chiropractors. West J Med 1989;150(3):351–5.

3   Sato A, Swenson RS. Sympathetic nervous system response to mechanical stress of the spinal column in rats. J Manip Physiol Ther 1984;7:141–7.

4   Budgell B, Hotta H, Sato A. Spinovisceral reflexes evoked by noxious and innocuous stimulation of the lumbar spine. JNMS 1995;3:122–31.

5   Daly JM, Frame PS, Rapoza PA. Sacroiliac subluxation: a common treatable cause of low-back pain in pregnancy. Fam Pract Res J 1991;11:149-59, reprinted in J Orth Med 1991;13(3):60–5.

6   Marshall P, Hamilton WG. Cuboid subluxation in ballet dancers. J Orthop Med 1994;16:90–5.

7   Rosner AL. The role of subluxation in chiropractic. Arlington, Virginia: Foundation for Chiropractic Education and Research, 1997.

8   Terrett AGJ. Misuse of the literature by medical authors in discussing spinal manipulative therapy injury. J Manip Physiol Ther 1995;18:203–10.

9   Sato A, Sato Y, Schmidt RF. The impact of somatosensory input on autonomic functions. Rev Physiol Biochem Pharm 1997;130.

10 Hasselberg PD. Chiropractic in New Zealand. Report of the commission of inquiry into chiropractic. Wellington, New Zealand: Government Printer, 1979.

CHAPTER 6

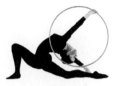

SCOPE OF PRACTICE

The term *scope of practice* has several meanings, and this chapter discusses:

- Legal scope of practice—what chiropractic practice is as defined by law in different states and countries.

- Diagnostic and treatment methods used in chiropractic practice.

- Conditions treated—who uses chiropractic services.

- Preventive care and health promotion.

- Frequency and duration of care—how often should you be treated and for how long?

A. Legal Scope of Practice

The legally defined scope of practice of chiropractic is not exactly the same in every country, state or province, but always has these common features:

1. Primary contact or care—meaning patients can consult a chiropractor directly without any requirement of medical referral.

2. The right and duty to perform a diagnosis, including the right to perform and/or order diagnostic skeletal x-rays. (In the U.S. the majority of chiropractors have x-ray facilities in their own offices, in Canada about 30% have x-ray facilities. Chiropractors choosing not to have their own x-ray machines order x-rays either from chiropractic specialist radiology clinics, medical radiology clinics or hospitals.)

3. The right to use spinal manipulation and a range of other manual and physical therapeutics.

4. No use of prescription drugs or surgery.

The legal scope of practice may appear in one or more of three levels of legislation—firstly the statute (e.g. The Chiropractic Act), secondly regulations or rules under that statute enacted by government, or thirdly in practice standards issued by the chiropractic board or regulatory authority established under the statute.

In some countries, there is no legal definition of scope of practice, which is the case in the U.K., Australia and New Zealand. In these circumstances the medical law or statute provides that the use of prescription drugs and surgery is restricted to the medical profession, and the chiropractic statute is silent on scope of practice. The benefits of this are that it avoids a political compromise on a legal definition of what the scope of practice of a profession is, reduces turf fights between health care professions and avoids a legal definition that becomes out of date as a profession grows or evolves. The legal definitions of chiropractic in the various U.S. states and Canadian provinces illustrate these problems.

Here are example scope of practice statements from different jurisdictions:

1. *U.S. Scope of Practice of Chiropractic Statements—Broad.*
   California: As taught in chiropractic colleges, without the use of drugs or surgery.

   Illinois: The treatment of human ailments without the use of drugs and without operative surgery.

2. *U.S.—Detailed*
   Pennsylvania: A branch of the healing arts dealing with the relationship between the articulations of the vertebral column, as well as other articulations, and the neuromusculoskeletal system and the role of these relationships in the restoration and maintenance of health. The term shall include systems of locating misaligned or displaced vertebrae of the human spine and other articu-

Methods of Diagnosis

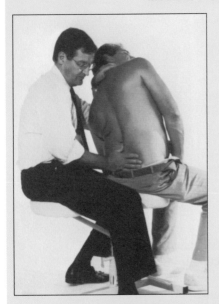

left and right: **Motion palpation of the lumbar spine and cervical spine to test for ranges of joint movement and spring end-feel.**

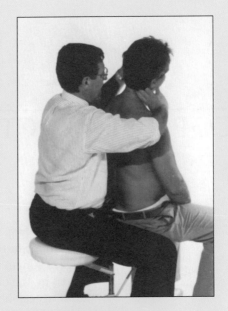

right: **Assessment of joint play movement in the thoracic spine—counter-rotation between the 4th and 5th thoracic vertebra (T4 and T5). The circles in the diagram indicate the placement of thumb contacts.**

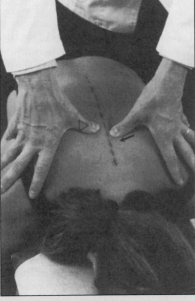

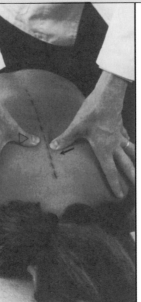

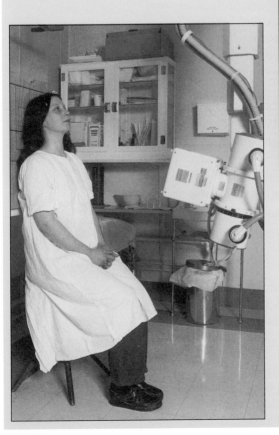

left and right: **Spinal x-rays and other imaging are an important part of chiropractic diagnosis with many patients. Imaging gives important structural information which can help determine which techniques to use, and which can rule out underlying problems that are contraindications to chiropractic manipulation.**

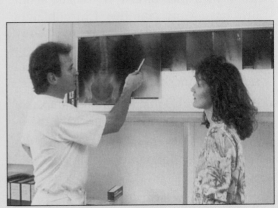

lations, the examination preparatory to the adjustment or manipulation of such misaligned or displaced vertebræ and other articulations; the furnishing of necessary patient care for the restoration and maintenance of health; and the use of Board approved scientific instruments of analysis, including x-ray. The term shall also include diagnosis, provided that such diagnosis is necessary to determine the nature and appropriateness of chiropractic treatment; the use of adjunctive procedures in treating misaligned or dislocated vertebræ or articulations and related conditions of the nervous system; and nutritional counselling, provided that nothing herein shall be construed to require licensure as a chiropractor in order to engage in nutritional counselling. The term does not include the practice of obstetrics or gynecology, the reduction of fractures or major dislocations, or the use of drugs or surgery.

3. *U.S.—Archaic (out of date)*
   Delaware: Chiropractic is the science of locating and removing any interference with the transmission of nerve energy. A license granted under the provisions of this chapter shall not entitle the licensee to use drugs, surgery, osteopathy, obstetrics, dentistry, optometry or podiatry.

4. *All U.S. states—Scope of Practice.* A summary of these and other licensure requirements can be obtained from an annual Official Directory published by the Federation of Chiropractic Licensing Boards (FCLB) 901 54th Avenue, Suite 101, Greely, CO 80634 USA, tel: 970-356-3500, fax: 970-356-3599, email: fclb@fclb.org, website: www.fclb.org.

5. *Canada—Typical and Contemporary*
   Newfoundland: Chiropractic means a professional service usually performed by a chiropractor directed towards the diagnosis, examination and treatment, principally by hand, and without use of drugs or surgery, of the spinal column, pelvis, extremities and associated tissues.

6. *Outside North America*
   Cyprus: Chiropractic means the healing method which, by chiropractic adjustment and manipulation of the spinal column and other articulations of the human body and without use of drugs or surgery, deals with

the restoration and maintenance of health and includes the use of analytical instruments and the application of therapies and diagnostic procedures as prescribed by regulations.

Denmark: Chiropractic practice includes the diagnosis, prevention and chiropractic treatment of biomechanic functional disorders of the spine, the pelvis and the extremities.

Chiropractic assessment methods include joint and soft tissue palpation—assessment by hand of ranges of joint motion, muscle tone, trigger points, skin roll, connective tissue adhesions, movement that provokes pain, . . .

B. **Diagnostic and Treatment Methods**

1. **Diagnosis**. There are two stages to the diagnostic process in chiropractic practice:

   a) *A General or Differential Diagnosis.* This is performed to see whether the patient falls within the scope of chiropractic practice or should be referred to another health professional (e.g. family physician, medical specialist, physical therapist, podiatrist, psychologist, etc).

   Methods are similar to medical diagnosis and include physical examination, history, various orthopedic and neurologic tests, laboratory tests, x-ray, MRI or other imaging as necessary. Radiology is a significant area of chiropractic education and practice, similar to dentistry. A number of chiropractors progress to postgraduate specialist status as radiologists, and some have authored respected radiology texts.[1,2]

   Given the nature of chiropractic practice, which involves many patients with spinal pain often following trauma or significant degeneration, there is quite frequent use of plain film x-ray in chiropractic practice. There is much less use of laboratory diagnosis and advanced imaging.[3] A survey of chiropractic practice in the United States and Canada in the years 1985–1991 reported that 54% of back pain patients had plain film x-ray, but only about 4% had advanced imaging studies such as CT or MRI. Labo-

Treatment Methods

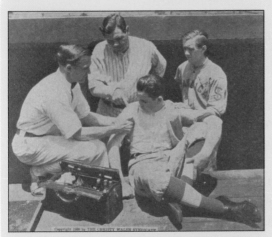

above: Erle Painter, DC, a chiropractor on the sports medicine team for the New York Yankees in the 1930s, here demonstrates a soft-tissue technique to Babe Ruth and others.

right: The rehabilitation clinic at Palmer College of Chiropractic circa 1945, showing a stationary bike long before this became standard gym equipment.

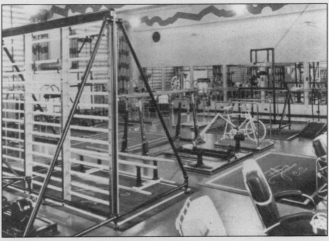

below: A modern chiropractic rehabilitation clinic.

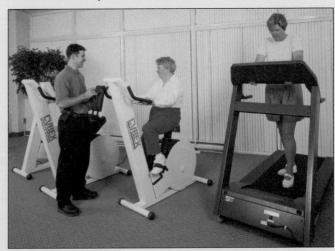

below: A chiropractor and patient in position for a lumbar spinal adjustment or manipulation.

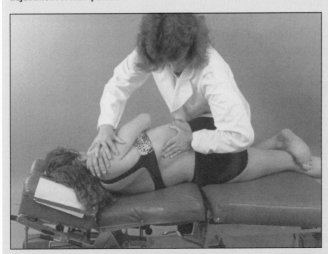

below: A modern chiropractic adjusting table incorporating motorized traction.

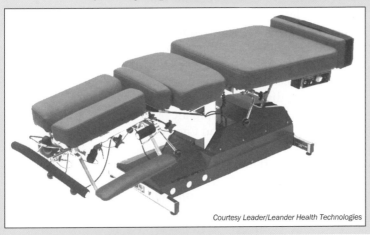

Courtesy Leader/Leander Health Technologies

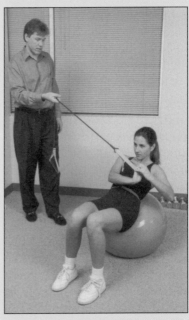

above: Muscle strengthening and balancing exercise using ball and resistance tubing.

ratory diagnosis tests were ordered for only 1% of patients.[4]

b) *A Specific Biomechanical and Chiropractic Analysis.* This is performed to assess joint, muscle and other soft-tissue restriction or dysfunction and related neurological effects. Chiropractic assessment methods include:

- Joint and soft tissue palpation—assessment by hand of ranges of joint motion, muscle tone, trigger points, skin roll, connective tissue adhesions, movement that provokes pain, etc.

- Range of motion measurement

- Postural symmetry

- Dynamic spinal loading

- Reactive leg length discrepancy

- Gait analysis

- Muscle imbalance tests

- Functional capacity and physical performance evaluations

2. **Treatment Methods**. The three main aspects of chiropractic management are manual treatments, prescription of preventive and rehabilitative exercises and patient education on matters such as posture, ergonomics, diet, healthy lifestyle, etc. More specifically:

a) *Manual Treatments:* These include joint adjustment, manipulation and mobilization; manual traction; trigger point therapy and other soft-tissue techniques. There is an emphasis on joint manipulation, a wide variety of quick, controlled techniques adapted for different joints that have been developed within chiropractic practice and education over several decades. The force applied is sudden rather than strong, and moves the joint through a small range of movement only—similar to the degree of joint movement when you "crack" a finger joint. (Manipulation, including its definition, mechanisms of action and effects are discussed fully in Chapter 7, "Manipulation.")

The traditional term for specific chiropractic techniques of manipulation is the chiropractic *adjustment*. The specialized forms of tables used by chiropractors, with various moving sections and mechanical features, are called *adjusting tables*.

To gain a full appreciation of the range of chiropractic adjusting or manipulative techniques for the various joints of the spine and skeleton, which have great variation anatomically, it is necessary to see one of the major technique texts, such as *Chiropractic Technique: Principles and Procedures* by Bergmann, Peterson

Table 1 Classification System for Chiropractic Manipulative/Adjustive Techniques

A. Manual Articular Manipulative and Adjustive Procedures
  1. Specific Contact Thrust Procedures
     a. High-velocity thrust
     b. High-velocity thrust with recoil
     c. Low-velocity thrust
  2. Nonspecific Contact Thrust Procedures
  3. Manual Force, Mechanically Assisted Procedures
     a. Drop-tables and terminal point adjustive thrust
     b. Flexion-distraction table adjustment
     c. Pelvic block adjusting
  4. Mechanical Force, Manually-Assisted Procedures
     a. Fixed stylus, compression wave adjustment
     b. Moving stylus instrument adjustment

B. Manual Nonarticular Manipulative and Adjustive Procedures
  1. Manual Reflex and Muscle Relaxation Procedures
     a. Muscle energy techniques
     b. Neurologic reflex techniques
     c. Myofascial ischemic compression procedures
     d. Miscellaneous soft-tissue techniques
  2. Miscellaneous Procedures
     a. Neural retraining techniques
     b. Conceptual approaches

Adapted from Guidelines for Chiropractic Quality Assurance and Practice Parameters, Haldeman S, et al. eds., Aspen, 1993

Table 2 Example Chiropractic Technique Systems

Full-spine high-velocity techniques	**Lumbo-pelvic techniques**
Diversified	Cox flexion-distraction
Gonstead	Leander
Thompson Terminal Point	Logan Basic
Pierce-Stillwagon	
Pettibon	
Chiropractic Biophysics	
Upper cervical techniques	**Miscellaneous/Instrument Adjustment**
Upper Cervical Specific	Sacro-Occipital Technique
NUCCA	Applied Kinesiology
Grostic	Activator
Orthogonal	Toftness

Adapted from Chiropractic in the United States: Training, Practice and Research, Cherkin, DC, Mootz, RD, eds., 1997.

and Lawrence.[5] Table 1 lists the classification scheme used in the recent development of American and Canadian chiropractic practice guidelines. Table 2 gives examples of specific chiropractic technique systems.

b) *Other Physical Treatments.* These include the use of heat, ice and electrotherapies (e.g. ultrasound, interferential therapy, TENS, etc.).

c) *Exercise and Rehabilitation.* The prescription of corrective, rehabilitative

... whatever the patient's condition, chiropractors fundamentally see themselves as diagnosing and treating the underlying joint and soft tissue dysfunction. This will have reflex effects in the nervous system that may influence various conditions and general health, not just the patient's primary complaint.

and preventive exercises is a second major aspect of chiropractic practice. This ranges from provision and supervision of recommended exercises, which is standard for all chiropractors, to operation of sophisticated multidisciplinary rehabilitation facilities. Chiropractic and medical rehabilitation protocols, as one would expect, are very similar. Chiropractic texts in this field, such as Liebenson's *Rehabilitation in Chiropractic Practice,*[6] include chapters by authors from medicine, physical therapy, osteopathy, exercise physiology, etc. Medical texts, such as Hochschuler's *Rehabilitation of the Spine,*[7] include chapters by chiropractors.

d) *Patient Education.* This is in specific areas, such as postural advice on lifting, sitting, sleeping and work postures, or

general education on nutrition and healthy lifestyle strategies. Chiropractic education includes course content in these areas and, in the U.S. national survey already mentioned, more than two-thirds of chiropractors reported using nutritional and general exercise counselling in practice.[3]

C. Conditions Treated by Chiropractors

1. **Introduction.** Various studies, which include national surveys in the U.S., Canada, Australia, and Europe, indicate that 95% of chiropractic patients have neuromusculoskeletal pain (NMS disorders), and fully 65-70% have back pain. The breakdown of all patient complaints seen in chiropractic practice, also illustrated in Figure 1, is:

Back pain		
• Low-back pain	65%	
• Mid-back pain	5%	70%
Other NMS pain		
• Head/neck pain	15%	
• Extremity pain	10%	25%
(shoulder, arm, leg, etc)		
Non-NMS pain		5%
• e.g. allergies, asthma, digestive disorders, menstrual problems, vision/hearing/balance disorders, etc).		
Total		100%

These figures need to be interpreted with some caution for several reasons. Firstly, third party payment policies influence what chiropractors record in their patient charts. For example, in the U.S., Medicare and some private insurers require chiropractors to report a musculoskeletal diagnosis as a condition of coverage.

Secondly, the realities of practice mean that many of the non-musculoskeletal complaints managed by chiropractors are secondary to musculoskeletal pain. This is illustrated by the case of Mrs. M discussed in Chapter 5 (see page 62). The patient was a motor vehicle accident victim who consulted a chiropractor for neck pain but also received relief for high blood pressure and edema. The primary complaint in her case was recorded as neck pain.

Thirdly, in many cases it is quite unclear whether the primary problem is musculoskeletal or non-musculoskeletal. As an example, chiropractors experience cases where a patient has a medical diagnosis of a

Figure 1 **Conditions Treated in Chiropractic Practice**

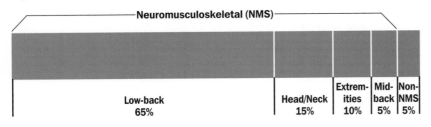

Neuromusculoskeletal (NMS)				
Low-back 65%	Head/Neck 15%	Extremities 10%	Mid-back 5%	Non-NMS 5%

cardiac problem but also has pronounced spinal dysfunction. Each condition influences or aggravates the other, and it is unclear which is of primary importance. Manual treatments to relieve the spinal dysfunction can completely resolve the pain being treated by the cardiologist as a pure cardiac disorder. A chiropractor, in these circumstances, feels it is more appropriate to record this in chiropractic clinical records as a case of joint and muscle dysfunction in the thoracic spine (mid-back) rather than a case of cardiac or chest pain. (Medical specialists report cases like this too.[8,9])

Fourthly, whatever the patient's condition, chiropractors fundamentally see themselves as diagnosing and treating the underlying joint and soft tissue dysfunction. This will have reflex effects in the nervous system that may influence various conditions and general health, not just the patient's primary complaint. To illustrate this point:

- In a national survey of over 5,000 U.S. chiropractors by the National Board of Chiropractic Examiners published in 1993, for which chiropractors were asked to list conditions routinely, often, and sometimes seen in their practices, the most common response was "joint dysfunction/spinal subluxation." Back pain was seldom mentioned, let alone non-musculoskeletal disorders.

- Chiropractors report clinical success in treating children with chronic ear infections (otitis media). It seems that some children have joint and muscle restrictions in the cervical spine, that correction of these may have a related effect on the function of the Eustachian tubes (probably their diameter and inclination), and that this improves drainage of the tubes and helps prevent future infections. The child's mother or father sees this as treating otitis media. A chiropractor generally describes this as treating joint and soft tissue dysfunction.

Bearing in mind all these considerations it remains clear, however, that the management of conditions thought by patients to be non-musculoskeletal is a relatively small part of chiropractic practice—about 5%. This percentage can be expected to gradually increase now that the areas of back and neck pain have given medical and chiro-

practic doctors a secure basis for working together. This means that many more medical physicians will be exposed to patients who experience non-musculoskeletal health benefits, and will then provide the patients for interdisciplinary clinical research to more fully investigate and understand the contribution of spinal dysfunction to problems such as cardiac disorders, respiratory disorders, dysmenorrhea and chronic constipation.

2. **Back Pain**. Management of back pain patients is the essential basis of chiropractic practice and the success of the profession. It is also a major area of cost to individuals and society, and one in which there are significant recent developments in medical understanding and practice. For these reasons back pain is dealt with in a separate chapter—see Chapter 8, "Back Pain."

3. **Head and Neck Pain**. This is the second most common area of chiropractic practice, after back pain. The two conditions are discussed together because patients often have both, as for example after motor vehicle whiplash injuries, and both routinely involve manual treatment of the cervical spine (neck). The term *head pain* includes headache and facial pain.

    a) *Mechanisms of Action—How does manual care work*. Manual treatments to the neck, jaw (temporomandibular joint or TMJ) and cranium work in a similar way to treatment of the low-back—through a combination of mechanical

Figure 2 **Posterior View of Cervical Spine**

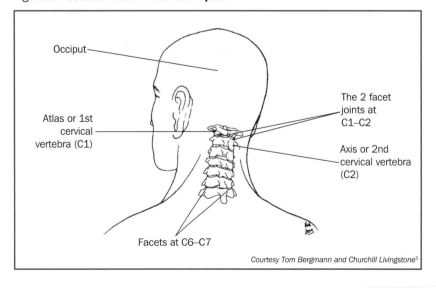

Courtesy Tom Bergmann and Churchill Livingstone[5]

and neurological effects. For a full discussion of this topic see Chapter 7, Section D, page 102. However there are two recent discoveries relating to the neck or cervical spine that are of particular interest:

i) *The importance of the facet joints of the cervical spine as a source of neck and head pain.* (See Figure 2 for an illustration of these joints.) Research by Bogduk, Lord and others has demonstrated the importance of these joints for neck pain and headache

There are three authoritative reviews in recent years that have concluded that neck manipulation and mobilization are safe, effective and appropriate for patients with various common forms of neck pain and headache.

conclusively. In the most recent trial, 60% of a group of patients with chronic neck pain and/or headache after whiplash were shown to have a specific facet joint as the source of the pain. The pain was relieved by injection of a local anesthetic into the joint, but not by injection of a neutral saline solution.[10]

The facet joints, found in pairs on the back of the cervical vertebrae, are rich in pain receptors. Chiropractic cervical manipulation is aimed primarily at gapping these facet joints to restore normal mechanics or movement.

ii) *The existence of bridges of connective tissue between the muscles and ligaments of the upper cervical spine and the dura at the base of the skull.* This is illustrated in the color plate opposite. This discovery by dental researchers in the U.S.[11] and chiropractic researchers in the U.K.[12] provides a much clearer anatomical basis for tension in the cervical spine as a cause of headache. The dura encloses the central spinal cord and is extremely pain sensitive. It is now known to be directly connected to muscles and ligaments in the neck.

b) *Safety and Effectiveness.* Some medical doctors express concern about the safety of neck manipulation. They tell their patients that manipulation is fine for the low-back "but don't let anyone manipulate your neck because there is a risk of stroke." You may have heard that. In recent years there have been a few media stories on the subject.

Is there established benefit from neck manipulation? What risks are involved? How does this compare with the risks of standard medical treatments for neck pain? What are the opinions of informed medical and other experts.?

There are three authoritative reviews in recent years that have addressed these questions, and all have concluded that neck manipulation and mobilization are safe, effective and appropriate for patients with various common forms of neck pain and headache. Each review has pointed out that there is less evidence of the benefits of manipulation for headache and neck pain than there is for back pain. On the other hand there is better evidence of effectiveness for manipulation than there is for common medical treatments for neck pain, including non-steroidal anti-inflammatory drugs (NSAIDS such as aspirin, ibuprofen, indomethacin) and other medication, and these medications have much higher risk rates than manipulation.

i) **Quebec Task Force Report.**[13] The first review was the report of the *Quebec Task Force on Whiplash Related Disorders* published in 1995. Leading medical researchers and clinicians from North America and Europe reviewed the literature and then provided treatment guidelines for whiplash injuries. Management of soft-tissue injuries to the neck (i.e. strain/sprain injuries with no bone fracture) should be similar to management of back pain—early return to function and activities rather than rest or immobilization in a collar, with joint manipulation and mobilization recommended to improve range of motion and reduce pain.

ii) **RAND Corporation Report.**[14] The second review was a RAND Corporation expert panel report in 1996 titled *The Appropriateness of Manipulation and Mobilization of the Cervical*

Connective Tissue Bridges Between Muscle and Dura in the Upper Cervical Spine.
A New Anatomical Basis for Cervical Headache and Chiropractic Treatment.

Courtesy of Dr. Gary Hack, Dr. Gwendolyn Dunn, Mi Young Toh
and Encyclopedia Britannica's 1998 Medical and Health Annual

Extract from the *Medical and Health Annual*

Does the new finding of a physical connection between skeletal muscle and the spinal dura represent the "missing link" that scientists have long sought to explain the pain of so-called muscle-contraction (tension) headaches?

Neurosurgeons describe the brain as "insensitive." It is known, however, that the covering of the brain, the dura, is extremely sensitive, and tension on the dura during neurosurgical procedures can produce pain experienced as headache. The Maryland scientists speculate that the newly described muscle–dura connection may transmit forces from neck muscles to the pain-sensitive dura.

A growing body of literature relates headaches to injury or pathology affecting neck structures. Moreover, a number of clinical trials

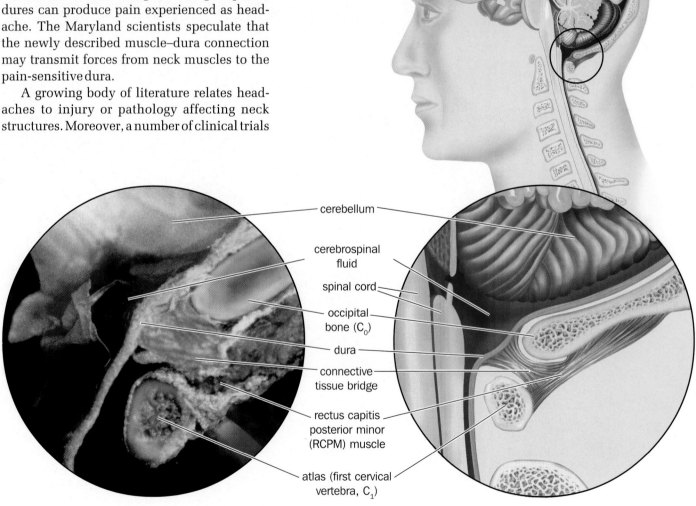

cerebellum

cerebrospinal fluid

spinal cord

occipital bone (C_0)

dura

connective tissue bridge

rectus capitis posterior minor (RCPM) muscle

atlas (first cervical vertebra, C_1)

Right: Illustration revealing a newly-discovered tissue bridge connecting the dura, the membranous covering of the brain and spinal cord, to the rectus capitis posterior minor (RCPM) muscle at the base of the skull between the atlas or first cervical vertebra and occipital bone or skull.

Left: Cadaver specimen showing the same structure.

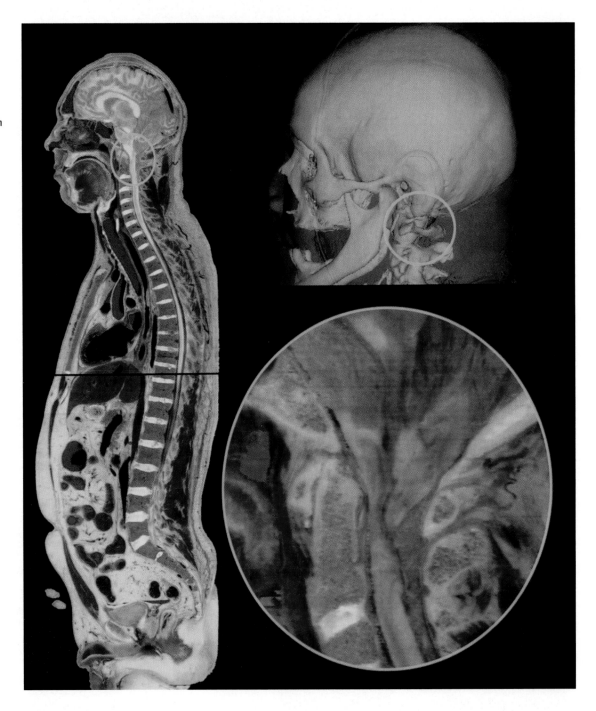

have suggested that treatments such as massage, spinal manipulation, and biofeedback directed at the neck are valuable for managing muscle-contraction headaches.

Spinal manipulation as a treatment for tension headache is predicated upon the assumption that dysfunction in the neck muscles contributes to the head pain; in the U.S. more than 90% of such procedures are performed by chiropractors. The muscle–dura connection may represent—at least in part—the underlying anatomic basis for the effectiveness of this treatment. Such treatment, as performed by a chiropractor, would decrease muscle tension and thereby reduce or eliminate pain by reducing the potential forces exerted on the dura via the muscle–dura connection.

Hack GD, Dunn G, Toh MY, *The Anatomist's New Tools*. Encyclopedia Britannica's 1998 Medical and Health Annual. *www.eb.com*.

Spine. In this report, as in many others RAND has done on the appropriateness of various medical treatments over the past 20 years, *appropriate care* is defined as the following:

"Expected health benefits to the patient (e.g. increased life expectancy, relief of symptoms, reduction of anxiety and improved functional capacity) exceeded expected health risks (e.g. mortality, morbidity, pain produced by the procedure) by a sufficiently wide margin that the procedure is worth doing."

In other words, on a balance of proven benefit and known risk rate, a treatment is or is not judged *appropriate.* The RAND expert panel, the nine members of which included two neurologists, a neurosurgeon, an orthopedic surgeon and primary care medical and chiropractic doctors, developed a list of 1,436 categories of neck pain and headache. Manipulation and mobilization were found appropriate for patients with many common categories of neck pain and headache where cervical signs of tenderness and limited range of motion were present.

There was a thorough review of comparative risk rates for manipulation and medical treatments, later summarized in the journal *Spine,*[15] and RAND reported the following serious complication rates:

- Cervical manipulation—1.5 per 1 million treatments (e.g. stroke from damage to a vertebral artery).

- Over-the-counter non-steroidal anti-inflammatory drugs (NS-AIDS)—1000 per 1 million patients, and 3200 per million for patients age 65 and above (e.g. serious gastrointestinal perforation or bleeding causing hospitalization and, for 10-20% of these patients, death).[16]

- Cervical spine surgery—15,600 per 1 million surgeries (e.g. paralysis or stroke).

Mortality rates are estimated at .27 per million for cervical manipulation (i.e. 1 in every 3–4 million treatments) but 6,900 per million for cervical spine surgery. In summary, there are cases of serious injury following neck manipulation but the risk is very small and remote compared with medical and surgical procedures given for the same health problems.

iii) **Cochrane Collaboration Systematic Review.** The third review was a systematic literature review by Aker, Gross, Goldsmith and Peloso, respectively a chiropractor, physiotherapist, epidemiologist and rheumatologist, published in the *British Medical Journal* in 1996 and titled Conservative Management of Mechanical Neck Pain: Systematic Overview and Meta-Analysis.[17] This research team from Canada has been accepted as the ongoing review team in the area of conservative management of the cervical spine within the Cochrane Collaboration, an international multidisciplinary network that is reviewing all the published health care trials in every field and making the results available on the Internet. This lends further strength to their conclusions which are:

- "Mobilisation is probably of at least short term benefit for patients with acute neck pain."

- "Manipulation is probably slightly more effective than mobilisation or physical therapy for some patients with sub-acute or chronic neck pain, and all three treatments are probably superior to usual medical care."

- "Manipulation and/or mobilisation may be beneficial for muscle tension headache."

- "More high quality research needs to be done before more definitive recommendations can be made regarding the use of manipulation or mobilisation for neck pain and headache."

The most authoritative review, recently published in *Spine,* suggests that those rare patients suffering significant harm from manipulation may have a connective tissue disease that weakens the ver-

Treatment of Extremity Joints

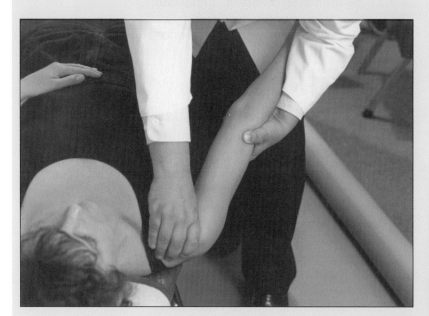

Adjustment techniques
for the shoulder, knee,
ankle and toe.

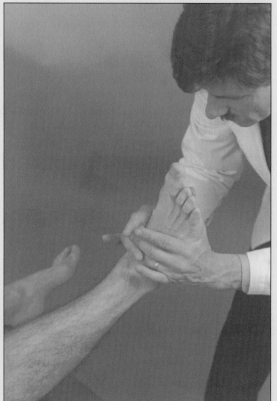

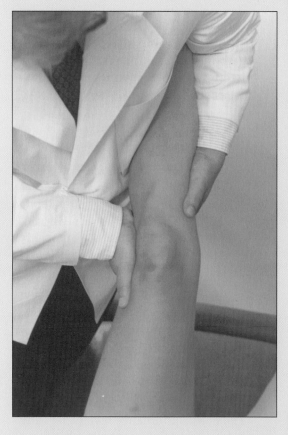

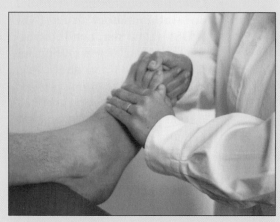

tebral arteries. This may be why many other common neck movements also lead to vertebral artery injury—kneeling at prayer, yoga, washing walls and ceilings, turning the head while driving or sneezing.[18]

c) ***Headache.*** This has been partly discussed already. These further points are made:

i) For research purposes the field of headache has been classified and defined by the International Headache Society (IHS). Major categories are migraine, tension-type headache and cervicogenic headache—headache "born in" or arising from the cervical spine. There are now formal controlled trials supporting the effectiveness of chiropractic management for each of these forms of headache.[19,20,21,22,23,24]

ii) There is still major disagreement between different health professionals, and between medical experts themselves, on the diagnosis, classification and treatment of headache. Treatment of most patients remains empirical—which simply means that the cause, proper diagnosis and treatment are all uncertain. The leading European neurologist Sjaastad has described the diagnostic confusion as "grave"[25] and the U.S. neurologist Saper explains that "the exact pathogenesis of migraine has yet to be established as differing views are held by a number of credible authorities."[26]

Most medical authorities on headache are neurologists who do not have the biomechanical training or interest to examine and investigate the neck. They usually look for causes inside the brain (intra-cranial causes). Many believe that headache is primarily caused by changes in brain chemistry that result in a lowering of the threshold at which pain is felt. Because of their training, chiropractors, now joined by an increasingly large number of medical specialists, argue that functional pathology in structures of the neck frequently plays a major role. Obviously

there are also many lifestyle and behavioral factors, from the food we eat to the levels of stress we endure.

iii) A recent survey from Denmark reports that cervicogenic headache as defined by the IHS is much more common that previously thought—at least as common as migraine.[27] Greater awareness of the significance of the cervical spine led in 1995 to medical and chiropractic researchers and clinicians forming the North American Cervicogenic Headache

Major categories of headache are migraine, tension-type headache and cervicogenic headache—headache "born in" or arising from the cervical spine.... A recent survey from Denmark reports that cervicogenic headache is at least as common as migraine.

Society (NACHS) "to continue the study of how neck pathology can cause headaches, so that this information becomes integrated into the mainstream of headache etiology and treatment." The NACHS's definition of cervicogenic headache is wider than that of the IHS, and is "referred pain perceived in any area of the head caused by a primary nociceptive (*i.e. pain producing*) source in the musculoskeletal tissues innervated by cervical nerves."

Many chiropractic patients express particular relief at being able to manage or cure chronic headache problems without the continued use and side effects of medication.

d) ***The Temporomandibular Joints (TMJs).*** These joints, joining the jaw to the skull and located just under and forward of the ears, are an often unsuspected cause of neck and facial pain and headache. It is quite common in chiropractic practice to have patients who have had extensive dental or medical care without relief, but whose problems resolve with a few manual treatments to the TMJ and associated muscle trigger points. Leading chiropractic texts in this area are by Darryl Curl, DC, DDS,[28] a chiropractor and dentist, and Steigerwald.[29]

4. **Extremities**. On average the treatment and prevention of biomechanical problems and pain in the shoulder, arms and legs—the extremities—represents approximately 10% of chiropractic practice. For some chiropractors specializing in sports chiropractic, extremity problems are the major area of practice—either prevention or treatment of injuries, or enhancement of performance. At the elite athlete level, optimum range and freedom of movement in the shoulder joints (swimmers) and sacroiliac, knee and ankle joints (runners) may be the difference

There are now trials showing that manipulation is effective for carpal tunnel syndrome, shoulder complaints, and knee problems.

between success and failure. This is the publicly expressed view of Donovan Bailey, the 100 meter world record holder and Olympic champion whose chiropractor travels with him, and many other athletes. Tiger Woods, the U.S. Olympic team, the Canadian swim team and the Australian Davis Cup team all have their chiropractors.

Extremity pain may be:

a) radiating or referred pain from a mechanical joint problem in the spine. Leg pain may be referred from a low-back disorder, and arm pain or numbness may be the result of a cervical spine dysfunction. This is illustrated in the photograph below.

b) from an extremity joint and/or associated soft tissues.

c) a combination of both, so that treatment of both areas is necessary for a successful result. An example is the "double crush" carpal tunnel syndrome, where wrist pain arises from restrictions in the wrist and cervical spine, and both areas need treatment.

There are now trials showing that manipulation is effective, for example, for carpal tunnel syndrome,[30,31,32] shoulder complaints,[33] and knee problems.[34] The trial of chiropractic manipulation for knee pain was done at the University of Calgary in Canada. Twenty-eight patients with knee pain and movement restriction who had not gained relief from medical rehabilitation and/or surgery were randomly sent to two groups—14 to a control group that received a chiropractic lower back functional assessment only and 14 to a treatment group that also received chiropractic manipulation of the sacroiliac joint. In the treatment group there was a significant reduction in muscle inhibition and knee joint restriction, whereas in the control group there was no significant change. For these patients the real cause of the knee problem was a related sacroiliac joint problem that was corrected by chiropractic adjustment.

5. **Non-Musculoskeletal Disorders**. This is the area of chiropractic practice that many medical doctors and members of the public find controversial. They can understand how chiropractic manipulation may be effective in relieving back and neck pain and headaches linked to tension in the cervical spine—but not why a chiropractor might treat a woman with dysmenorrhea and an infant with colic. And, because these problems seem unrelated to the spine and the chiropractic scope of practice, few patients with them seek chiropractic care.

Treatment of non-musculoskeletal conditions represents an economically insignificant part of chiropractic practice—indeed, practice in these areas by chiropractors has delayed their general acceptance by the medical profession and the public. For these reasons the chiropractic approach to non-musculoskeletal disorders is now explained with case examples and at greater length than management of musculoskeletal pain.

Arm or leg pain may be referred pain from a problem in the spine.

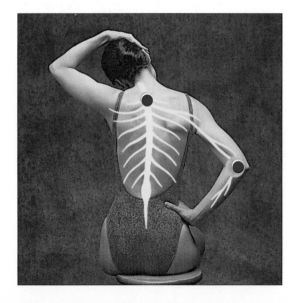

The basis of treatment has already been discussed under Chiropractic Principles (*see Chapter 5, "Principles and Goals of Chiropractic Care"*). Before case examples are given, these further background comments may be useful:

- All claims made by responsible members of the chiropractic profession on this subject are now also made by those who practice manipulation in the medical and osteopathic professions. They agree that restoring correct function to spinal joints and associated soft tissues by manipulation also produces reflex effects in the nervous system. These reflexes are transmitted through centers in the spinal cord that contain a common pool of nerves/neurons that regulate musculoskeletal function and visceral function. This means that spinal joint manipulation may have an effect on visceral functions and disorders and overall health and wellbeing. Exact effects are never certain. However they may be dramatic and of fundamental importance for individual patients.

John Mennell, MD, the leading figure in U.S. manual medicine during the past 30 years, wrote: "Pain from joint pathology may be appreciated in any distant structure which shares its nerve supply with the joint. Indeed, one may postulate interference with the function of viscera as a result of referred joint pain through a somatic/visceral reflex arc. I am certain that such phenomena occur."[35]

Alan Stoddard, MD, DO, the leading figure in English manual medicine and osteopathy during the same period, explains in his text that he has not dealt with individual diseases "because this would spoil the basic idea that whatever the disorder, the principle behind treatment is to restore proper and harmonious mechanics."[36] He adds:

"It is impossible to say whether (manipulation) is effective or not in any one disorder. So much depends in each case on the structural factors, the type of patient, and the competence of the practitioner, but it is still as true as ever, whatever the patient's disease, that he will have a better chance of recovery if he is mechani-

cally sound. . . . Mechanical lesions are ætiological in many diseases because the lesions weaken those viscera which are reflexly and segmentally linked with them. . . . To claim that mechanical lesions are the only factors in disease is, of course, ludicrous. They are rarely totally responsible, but they cannot and should not be discounted in any disease."[36]

- When chiropractic views in this area,

". . . whatever the patient's disease, he will have a better chance of recovery if he is mechanically sound. . . . Mechanical lesions are ætiological in many diseases because the lesions weaken those viscera which are reflexly and segmentally linked with them." —Alan Stoddard, MD DO

and medical criticisms, were fully reviewed by an independent Commission of Inquiry in New Zealand, the Commission found that "where there are organic and/or visceral symptoms chiropractic treatment may provide relief, but this is unpredictable, and in such cases the patient should be under concurrent medical care if that is practicable."[37] The Commission had heard and examined much patient testimony, some of which is referred to below.

The Commission's conclusion is not only endorsed by the chiropractic profession but is also what happens in practice. Patients who consult a chiropractor for hearing or vision problems, or visceral disorders such as respiratory, digestive or pelvic problems, almost invariably have prior or concurrent medical assessment and care. That is the way it should be, with the professions working together for improved understanding and results.

- There are few good clinical trials by anyone—medical, chiropractic, osteopathic or other researchers—in this field. From a chiropractic perspective this has been for two main reasons. Firstly, chiropractic resources have been directed to areas of more immediate clinical importance in daily practice, such as back pain and headache. Secondly, cooperation with medical researchers has been necessary to obtain the number of patients required. Now that such cooperation is possible, trials on conditions such as infantile colic and childhood asthma are being performed. Case reports, as already explained (Chapter 1), do not represent scientific proof. Rather they are the starting point, initial evidence worthy of consideration and then used as a basis for further study and research. The following discussion relies upon these.

"It was put to Mr. R in cross-examination that his son's asthmatic condition could have relieved itself naturally, . . . Mr. R rejected that suggestion and so do we; . . ."

a) ***Childhood Disorders***

i) ***Asthma***. Chiropractic patients frequently have good results with respiratory restrictions including asthma. Here is a case as reported by the New Zealand Commission of Inquiry into Chiropractic.

Mr. R's son

"One day Mr. R, a chiropractic patient who had suffered from a serious back problem for which he had obtained relief by chiropractic treatment, told his chiropractor that he was concerned about the condition of his son, not quite 2 years old, who was an asthmatic. The child was under medical specialist care, but he seemed to be getting worse. As Mr. R testified:

"By this time my son had developed a constant wheeze and was losing weight due to his inability to eat the right quantity of food, plus he was finding it very difficult to sleep at night due to the wheezing and shortness of breath.

"Mr. R and his wife had to take it in turns sitting with the little boy throughout the night in case the child woke up and needed attention.

"The chiropractor suggested that Mr. R bring the child in for examination. He did not promise a cure.

Following examination, the chiropractor suggested the child might have had a fall at some time (which was the case) and adjusted the child's neck. Immediately there was a dramatic improvement. Mr. R described it as miraculous. *We didn't even get out of the waiting room and his constant wheeze, which was pretty bad, had almost disappeared. On the night of the first treatment the child had his first uninterrupted sleep for some considerable time.*

"As we have said, Mr. R was intensively cross-examined, and we therefore had a full opportunity to assess what weight we could place on his evidence. The Commission was most impressed with him. It was clear that his son's instant response to the chiropractic treatment had left a deep impression on him. He did not expect any particular result, and that is why he spontaneously described the result as miraculous. He was reliving the moment as he told us that.

"It was put to Mr. R in cross-examination that his son's asthmatic condition could have relieved itself naturally, and (in effect) that the chiropractic treatment had nothing to do with it. Mr. R rejected that suggestion and so do we; we cannot accept that within minutes of the chiropractic treatment the boy's asthmatic symptoms remitted themselves purely by coincidence. We are driven to find that the major relief the child experienced within that short time was a direct result of the chiropractic treatment he received."[38]

There have now been three studies assessing chiropractic management of asthma in children.[39,40,41] These have reported mixed results, with stronger improvement in subjective measurements (relief from symptoms, reduced use of bronchio-dilators and medication) than objective measurements (peak air-flow rates). Many children experience excellent results but it remains unclear which children will get the best results and why. All children in the trials have had spinal joint dysfunction in the thoracic and/or cervical spine—there is obviously no basis for chiropractic treatment if there is no musculoskeletal restriction. It will not be hard for anyone to understand that an asthmatic child may have tension in the thoracic spine and rib cage. The issues are when and how this may be linked to asthma. (For fuller comment on how a spinal problem may cause asthma see page 84.)

ii) ***Bed wetting (enuresis).*** This is found in 20% of 4–5 year olds, twice as frequently in males as in females, and produces great distress. Causes are unclear. Explanations include behavioral, biological and psychological reasons, and often there will be more than one cause. There are many medical treatments—including periodic waking, fluid restriction, bell and pad, dry bed training, psychotherapy, hypnotherapy and chemotherapy—none supported by strong research.

Chiropractors often report successful results. An Australian study involving 171 children between the ages of 4 and 15 with relevant spinal dysfunction reported only moderate success, better than psychotherapy and periodic waking, but less than some reports of bell and pad and dry bed training methods.[42] The study has been criticized for looking at the effect of chiropractic manual treatments only, whereas in chiropractic practice these are generally combined with other methods such as fluid restriction and periodic waking.

A U.S. trial involving 57 children between the ages of 5 and 13 com-

pared active chiropractic care (spinal adjustment or manipulation at the level or levels of restricted range of motion) and a sham or placebo treatment (use of an adjusting device or hammer with a non-tension setting at a spinal level without restricted motion). Parents kept a diary with dry/wet measurements. After 12 weeks (10 weeks of treatment and then 2 of observation) results were variable. On one hand 7 or 25% of the children receiving chiropractic care had a 50% or greater reduction in wet night frequency from approximately 9 wet nights per 2 weeks to 4 or less per 2 weeks, whereas none of the sham or control patients had a 50% improvement. On the other hand, some children receiving active chiropractic care had little improvement and overall there was no statistically significant difference between the two groups. Those children improving tended to have spinal restrictions in both the pelvic and upper cervical spine areas.[43]

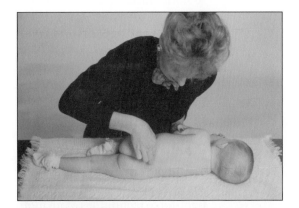

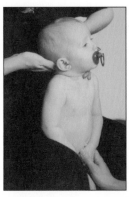

Treatment techniques for the low-back and cervical spine in infants.

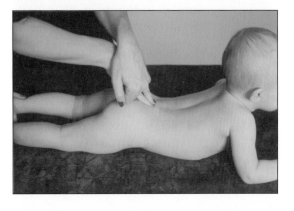

iii) ***Colic***. Infantile colic is a term used to describe persistent, often violent crying for no apparent reason in otherwise healthy and thriving young infants. The distress is believed to be a reaction to pain. Colic begins at 1–4 weeks of age and usually ends spontaneously at 3–4 months of age. The source of pain is unclear. Because of the high incidence of spinal joint restrictions in colicky infants, and the interactions between spinal and digestive dysfunction, chiropractors postulate that the pain may be aggravated or caused by the spinal problem.

Clinical experience of good results has now been supported by a multicenter study of 316 infants in Denmark.[44] To be entered into the study the infants, who had an average age of 5.7 weeks, had to have colic (normal weight gain and health but persistent crying for approximately 5 hours per day and an inability to be comforted by various normal means), spinal functional disturbance, and behavior during colic that included motoric unrest, such as frequent flexing of the knees towards the abdomen and/or backward bending of the head and trunk. Of 569 infants, 253 did not meet these criteria—in other words a precise diagnosis is important and only some infants with colic will be appropriate for chiropractic treatment.

Treatment, given an average of 3 times over 2 weeks, comprised light-force techniques of no more trouble to the infant than basic physical examination. There was a success rate of 94% (colic stopped—60%, significantly improved—34%) and the researchers concluded that, with appropriately selected infants, "standard chiropractic treatment constitutes an effective treatment for infantile colic." This was a prospective study, without a comparison or control group receiving medical or no care. The researchers called for a controlled trial and this is now nearing completion.

iv) ***Hearing Impairment***. Here is a further case independently assessed and reported by the New Zealand Commission:

Mrs. D's Daughter

"Mrs. D told us of chiropractic relief which had been given to her young daughter, who suffered from impaired hearing. Mrs. D and her husband took her to an ear, nose and throat specialist. The specialist thoroughly examined her and recommended surgery. Mrs. D was reluctant to agree to this course, and thought that chiropractic should at least be tried. Mrs. D had been to a chiropractor before for a back complaint. She and her husband took the child to the chiropractor who examined her and adjusted her spine in the area of the neck.

"Much to Mr. and Mrs. D's surprise, the child was able to hear a whisper from across the room the following day. In Mrs. D's words, recalling the child's previous condition, that to me was miraculous.

"They took the child back to the ear, nose and throat specialist. The specialist tested the child. He found, to his surprise, that her hearing had improved to a level of 100/98. That was a remarkable change. Her hearing had become normal. He asked what the parents had been doing. They told him they had taken the child to the chiropractor and his response, according to Mrs. D, was: of course if you are going to do this sort of thing you might get temporary relief but you will have her back here within 6 months.

"Mrs. D told us that that prediction had fortunately proved incorrect. Her daughter is now trained as a nurse and she has no problem. In fact, her hearing is a little bit too good sometimes. We have no reason to think, from seeing and hearing Mrs. D on the witness stand, that she was giving us other than an accurate and unemotional report."[37]

v) ***Lowered Resistance Generally***. The above categories deal with specific conditions. It has been explained that chiropractic principles, confirmed by clinical experience, suggest that restoring freedom of movement to spinal joints and muscles may improve overall function in a variety of ways. It has also been explained that medical and osteopathic doctors who practice manipulation have similar theories and experiences. Here is a case report from Gutmann, a German medical manipulator:

"History. An 18 month old boy with normal birth had early recurring tonsillitis, frequent enteritis, and therapy resistive conjunctivitis. The infant suffered often with colds, rhinitis, earache, and increasing sleeping problems. He was unable to remain in a sleeping position for prolonged periods and screamed during the night. Touching his neck triggered marked defensive movements and screams apparently due to pain. As a baby he had fallen off the changing table several times, including 2 weeks before the first fit.

" Manual and radiological examinations. Straightened cervical spine and atlas fixation (i.e. *restricted movement of the first vertebra)*.

"Treatment and Results. After the first manual thrust to the atlas the child asked to be put to bed and for the first time slept peacefully until morning. His previously disturbed appetite normalised completely. It was noted that the infant could run more securely and did not fall as frequently. His conjunctivitis cleared completely."[45]

vi) ***Otitis Media***. Otitis media (OM) is an inflammation of the middle ear. It is not a primary disease, but a complication of colds, sinusitis and sore throats. Obviously chiropractic treatment has no role in treatment of acute OM, but it can be most successful in the prevention of chronic, recurring OM. In a recent U.S. case report by Phillips,[46] a 2 year old girl suffered chronic OM in both ears despite several regimens of antibiotics and tympanostomy tube insertions in both ears. Her parents saw no improvement in symptoms, which included sore throats, nausea, poor appetite, ear pain and ear discharge, following the tube surgery. Six months later they consulted a chiropractor.

Palpation revealed that the atlas or first cervical vertebra was fixed on the right side. A first manual treatment to restore normal range of motion produced significant reduction in ear discharge and pain over the next 3 days. Further treatments brought complete relief. There were acute recurrences 5 and 6 months later, which cleared within the week after cervical mobilization. On follow-up over a period of 4 years the young girl remained symptom free.

The likely explanation for these results is that restoring motion to the cervical spine and altering its neurophysiology improves the drainage of the Eustachian tubes in the ears—probably by altering the inclination and/or the diameter of the tubes. For two series of cases reporting more fully on the benefits of chiropractic treatment and the factors involved, the first of which followed 332 children with otitis media, see studies by Fallon[47] and Froehle.[48] The first full trial of chiropractic treatment is now underway in the U.S. and is comparing three groups of patients—one receiving chiropractic management, a second medical management, and a third combined chiropractic and medical management.

vii) **Tonsillitis**. As with otitis media, chiropractic treatment may be effective for children who have chronic recurring infections and cervical spine dysfunction. The largest published case series is by Lewit, a Czech neurologist and manual medicine specialist.[49] Working with a throat specialist he noted a high frequency of up-

Palmer, the founder of chiropractic, claimed that his first patient had his hearing restored by manipulation of the thoracic spine. Bourdillon, a medical manipulator from Canada, has reported a similar experience.

per cervical spine dysfunction in children with chronic relapsing tonsillitis. In a group of 76 children, 70 had "dysfunction between the occiput and the atlas" (i.e. between the head and the first vertebra)."

Thirty-seven were given manipulation and then followed for 5 years. Two out of three (25 or 67.6%) were cured. Twenty-five had tonsillectomy operations. Of these, 3 out of 4 (19 or 76%) still suffered movement restrictions which were then treated with manipulation. Lewit concluded that "tonsillitis goes hand in hand with movement restriction in the craniocervical junction . . . with little tendency to spontaneous recovery and the danger of permanently disturbed function in one of the most sensitive regions of the locomotor system" and that "our experience suggests that blockage at this level increases the susceptibility to recurrent tonsillitis."

b) **General Disorders**. Chiropractic management has been reported as effective for the relief of various conditions apparently remote from the spine. It is important to repeat the principle behind treatment of patients with these conditions, some

of which are now discussed. It is not that these conditions are themselves an indication of chiropractic care; rather, it is that some patients with these conditions may have related spinal dysfunction that is a significant cause of the patient's problem, sometimes the most significant cause. (For further comment, including support for the principle from medical specialists, see page 77.)

i) **Hearing/Vision/Equilibrium Disorders**.

Hearing: Daniel David Palmer, the founder of chiropractic, claimed that his first patient had his hearing restored by manipulation of the thoracic spine. Bourdillon, a medical manipulator from Canada and author of the text *Spinal Manipulation*, has reported a similar experience.[50] In summary:

- A man aged 35 had an accident in which "his head was driven downwards so that the neck was telescoped into the chest." This caused severe pain in the upper thoracic spine and then a month later development of "Ménière's Syndrome consisting of unilateral deafness, tinnitus (ringing of the ears) and vertigo so severe that he almost always vomited and the only relief he obtained was by going to bed." After 18 months, and much unsuccessful investigation and treatment, he sought assessment and treatment by a medical doctor practicing spinal manipulation.

- He was first treated by cervical manipulation of the restricted neck joints but "relief was transient and very far from complete."

- When the thoracic spine was examined a biomechanical lesion at the T4-5 joint was found and "manipulative treatment to this joint resulted in dramatic and lasting relief of all symptoms referred to, including the deafness."

Bourdillon concludes that Palmer's claim to have restored a patient's hearing by manipulation of the upper thoracic spine "may not be quite as fantastic as it sounds" even though their common experience is hard to explain on known anatomy and physiology.

At chiropractic meetings one hears a number of anecdotal accounts of improved or restored hearing, though such cases are uncommon and the indication for possible chiropractic management is spinal fixation or restriction rather than impaired hearing. (For a similar case involving a child, see page 80.)

Vision: Similar cases are reported for visual impairment. Gilman and Bergstrand,[51] respectively an optometrist and chiropractor, describe an elderly man who suffered complete loss of vision following head injury. He fell between two logs hitting his head, immediately experienced head pain and dizziness, and awoke blind the next day.

He first consulted an optometrist and then an ophthalmologist. A CT scan ruled out cerebral blood clot or other pathology as a cause and, after 3 months, the diagnosis was blindness due to head trauma. Vision loss was thought to be permanent, with no treatment indicated. The optometrist, who had experience of vision changes after chiropractic treatment in other cases, referred the patient for chiropractic evaluation. This revealed fixation in the upper cervical spine.

The patient received 11 treatments of chiropractic adjustment or manipulation to the upper cervical joints over a 3 month period. Vision improvement, which was monitored throughout by the referring optometrist, started after the third treatment. There was progressive improvement over 6 weeks to normal vision and ability to read comfortably. The authors rule out spontaneous remission and postulate two mechanisms to explain the results—restoring blood supply to the optic nerve (by removing interference with

> ..."it is important to stress that a cervical factor may be present in all forms of vertigo and dizziness ... in no field is manipulation more effective than in the treatment of disturbances of equilibrium."
> —Karel Lewit, MD

the sympathetic innervation of the blood vessels of the optic nerve), or removing interference with other nerve pathways to the ophthalmic artery and the eye (via the first four cervical nerves, the rami communicans, the superior cervical ganglion, the cavernous plexus, the ciliary ganglion, the oculomotor nerve, and the ophthalmic branch of the trigeminal nerve).

Cases such as this may become more frequent now that it is more common for medical specialists and chiropractors to work together cooperatively. The Australian ophthalmologist Gorman, working with chiropractors, has now reported 18 cases where visual field loss has been restored following spinal manipulation.[52,53]

Equilibrium: Chiropractic management has a more established role in the treatment of dizziness and vertigo. In the largest controlled study Fitz-Ritson reports a complete success rate with 90% of 112 acute and chronic patients by using a range of manual techniques and exercises.[54] Bracher et al report similar results with 16 patients with cervical vertigo referred for chiropractic care by medical specialists.[55] Lewit comments, "it is important to stress that a cervical factor may be present in all forms of vertigo and dizziness...in no field is manipulation more effective than in the treatment of disturbances of equilibrium."[56]

Vertigo may be *central* (i.e. in the central nervous system—the brain, brainstem or spinal cord)

One of the most common non-musculoskeletal disorders for which patients seek chiropractic care is asthma....spinal manipulation removes the physical restriction and/or neurological imbalance that is an underlying cause of the body's over-sensitivity in some patients.

and/or *cervical* (i.e. a problem in the muscles, joints and ligaments of the neck, irritating nerves and the vertebral arteries and altering incoming information to the central nervous system). Fitz-Ritson reviews the three mechanisms for cervical vertigo—cervical sympathetic irritation, abnormal neck reflexes, and mechanical compression or irritation of the vertebral artery—all of which are "well-supported clinically and experimentally." However they are often overlooked in medical practice because medically trained specialists assume a central cause.

Hypertension. A case example has already been given of relief from moderate, long-standing hypertension, or high blood pressure, following chiropractic treatment (see Chapter 5, page 63). Yates and Lamping, in a trial comparing one group of patients receiving chiropractic manipulation and a control group receiving a sham treatment, have demonstrated a significant reduction in hypertension in the treatment group.[57] This trial is too small to represent convincing evidence and more research is necessary.

ii) ***Respiratory/Digestive/Cardiac Disorders***

Respiratory*:* One of the most common non-musculoskeletal disorders for which patients seek chiropractic care—and often receive quite dramatic results—is asthma. The New Zealand Commission, after hearing from 188 such patients, and a medical witness who commonly referred selected patients with asthma for chiropractic assessment and treatment, described relief from asthma as one of the more consistent and frequent benefits of chiropractic treatment.[58]

How could spinal manipulation and other chiropractic treatments help with asthma? This is a question that many readers will have—not only with respect to asthma but with other conditions apparently remote from the spine. Let's therefore pause to discuss this in more detail.

Asthma is a chronic lung condition that is characterized by difficulty in breathing. In a person with asthma, the airways narrow, requiring the person to breathe with more effort to move air in and out of the lungs. The narrowing is the result of inflammation of the tissues lining the walls of the airways, spasm of the smooth muscles and secretion of mucous into the airways. There are numerous factors that may cause this. They are not all well understood, and the factors are different for each patient.

An immediate cause of asthma may be over-sensitivity (hyperreactivity) to certain stimuli such as certain foods, cigarette smoke, pollen, dust mites, exercise, mould or a respiratory viral infection that produces inflammation. Underlying causes—the reasons for the over-sensitivity—may be chemical or neurological imbalances in the body. The theoretical basis for benefit from chiropractic manipulation is that it corrects a physical and neurological imbalance, in this way:

- Restricted movement of one or more spinal joints irritates nerves at the spinal and nerve-root levels. (The chiropractic term for this is subluxation.)

- This mechanical and neurological disturbance affects chest wall function, alters airway tone and does this directly or by means of neurogenic inflammation.

- Correction of subluxation by spinal manipulation restores normal mechanical and nerve function—it removes the physical restriction and/or neurological imbalance that is an underlying cause of the body's over-sensitivity in some patients.

(For fuller details see the review *Asthma and Chiropractic* by Bronfort.[41])

Chiropractic management is based on spinal manipulation but includes review of diet, identification of allergens and general advice. Studies by Miller[59] and Hviid[39] reported changed vital capacity and peak expiratory flow rates in asthmatic patients following manipulation, but studies by Bronfort[60] and Balon[40] have suggested subjective improvement only. Patients felt better and were less reliant on medication but there was no objective change in peak expiratory flow rates.

Asthma can be life-threatening and obviously most patients should be under medical care. What all the evidence suggests, however, is that chiropractic co-management is safe, generally beneficial, dramatically effective for some patients and that therefore chiropractic assessment for

spinal contributing factors should often be considered. Patients will want to choose medical and chiropractic doctors who can work cooperatively. Future research will undoubtedly better identify those classes of patients most likely to respond to chiropractic treatment. (For specific comment on childhood and adolescent asthma see page 78.)

Digestive*:* Many patients report

Many patients report relief from chronic constipation following manipulation of the low-back.

relief from chronic constipation following manipulation of the low-back, usually for a primary complaint of back pain. In many cases, the constipation existed for months or years before the back pain problem, but resolved when normal function was restored in the lumbar spine. Other patients receiving manipulation for dysfunction in the mid-back (thoracic spine) find relief from various other digestive disorders. There are now three studies reporting that manipulation can help the remission or healing of duodenal ulcer.[61,62,63] The most recent, by medical researchers Pikalov and Vyatcheslav at the Moscow Central Hospital, involved patients with acute spinal dysfunction and uncomplicated duodenal ulcer confirmed by endoscopic examination.

In this study, one group received standard drug therapy and dietary regime over 4 to 7 weeks. Another group received 3 weeks of spinal manipulation and the same dietary regime. The main result measured was full clinical remission of the ulcer, either by epithelialization (smooth healing of the lining of the duodenum) or cicatrization (healing by scar formation). Healing took an average of 16.4

days in the manipulation group—
10 days and 40% faster than the
average 25.7 days in the medical
group. Initial size of the ulcers
was equivalent in both groups.
The result was statistically significant.

Cardiac: With respect to cardiac
disorders, consider the following
example:

- Mr. AT, a middle-aged mechanic complaining of chest
  pain, is referred by his family
  physician to a cardiologist.
  Examinations reveal many
  classic signs and symptoms of
  myocardial ischemia—deep
  chest and arm pain, paleness,
  sweating, cardiac dysrhyth-
  mia and coronary arterioscle-
  rosis. He is told he has a heart
  problem, must stop strenuous
  work and is prescribed ni-
  trates and then beta-blockers.
  Nothing seems to help the
  chest pain.

- Anxious to find anything that
  might help, and feeling tight-
  ness in his mid back, he con-
  sults a chiropractor. Examination reveals joint restrictions
  and muscle tension in the
  lower cervical and thoracic
  spine. Palpation of the top two
  segments of the thoracic spine
  reproduces the cardiac pain.
  X-rays show marked narrowing of the intervertebral foramen at C6/C7. After a short
  course of spinal manipulation
  joint function is normal and
  the pain is fully relieved. Others signs and symptoms are
  also resolved.

A chiropractic case similar to this
was presented before the New
Zealand Commission. The above
case, however, comes from a paper titled *Functional Disorders of
Internal Organs due to Vertebral
Lesions* by the German cardiologist Kunert.[64] In this paper Kunert
presents patients medically diagnosed as having heart disease or
respiratory block but found at his
hospital unit primarily to have
vertebral dysfunction. He concludes:

"We have records of numerous
cases similar to the one described
here, in which a definite connection appears to exist between a
functional disorder in an internal
organ and a spinal lesion . . .
lesions of the spinal column are
perfectly capable of simulating,
accentuating, or making a major
contribution to (organic) disorders. There can, in fact, be no
doubt that the state of the spinal
column does have a bearing on the
functional status of the internal
organs."

Logically, there are four possible
explanations for cases such as
these—and in all of them it is
important to the patient that there
be chiropractic and medical
examinations and interdisciplinary understanding and cooperation. Firstly, the spinal problem
may be simulating or mimicking
heart disease. Some pathology is
present but is not the cause of the
problem. This is analogous to the
well-known situation in which a
patient has clear evidence of a
herniated lumbar disc but this is
not in fact the cause of his back
and leg pain—this pain is relieved
by manipulation of the lumbar
spine, even though the herniation
remains.

Secondly, heart disease and pain
have caused a reflex reaction in
the spine and paraspinal muscles.
The resulting spinal dysfunction
then exaggerates or mimics cardiac pain.

Thirdly, heart disease caused the
spinal dysfunction as just mentioned, the underlying disease
has now gone, but the spinal problem continues to give symptoms
simulating the former heart disease.

Fourthly, the spinal dysfunction is a significant cause of the heart disease, through altered somato-visceral reflexes. Animal model experiments have confirmed that mechanical stimulation of the spinal nerves produces such reflexes that do influence cardiac function,[65,66] but the exact clinical effects of these reflexes remain unknown. Pain is also a stress factor, so an effect on visceral function from spinal pain is understandable from this perspective too.

iii) ***Pelvic Disorders/Dysmenorrhea***. Speaking at an interdisciplinary research meeting for chiropractors and physicians in London in 1987, John O'Brien, an English orthopedic surgeon, observed that in his experience thousands of British women would be spared hysterectomy operations each year if they first had a chiropractic assessment—the true cause of their problem was often referred pain from the lumbar spine that could have been successfully treated with chiropractic manipulation.

A variety of urological, gynecological, sexual and bowel disorders may be managed successfully under chiropractic care. Browning reviews the literature and reports on 10 cases from his practice.[67] The most detailed case report follows.

- This involves a 41 year old married woman who first experienced low-back and abdominal pain as a child which was diagnosed as constipation. Over the next 30 years she experienced continuing and increased back pain and radiating pain to the left leg and had severe low-back pain through four pregnancies.

- From about age 20 the patient experienced increasing uro-

logical, gynecological, sexual and bowel disorders over a 20 year period. These were all major problems when the patient consulted a chiropractor, Browning. For example, for 2 years the patient could only commence and maintain bladder function by "self-administered deep bladder massage." Bowel evacuation was only possible once every

> ***"... thousands of women would be spared hysterectomy operations each year if they first had a chiropractic assessment."***
> —John O'Brien, MD

4–5 days, and then with difficulty and use of a laxative or suppository. Pain on intercourse had led to loss of sexual desire and inability to achieve orgasm.

- After physical, x-ray and laboratory examination the chiropractic diagnosis was "a centrally located lumbar disc lesion with resultant left L5, S1, S2, S3 and right S2 and S3 nerve root compression."

- Treatment, which was directed at reducing the nerve root compression caused by the lumbar disc lesion, comprised closed reduction distractive decompression, lumbar curve reducing exercises, a lumbosacral orthopedic appliance and bed rest.

- Results were highly significant, both for the pain and the organic dysfunctions. After two weeks of care, bladder control and bowel function returned to normal, following years of serious dysfunction. The sexual difficulties also resolved completely.

Finally, with respect to dysmenorrhea, chiropractic researchers Kokjohn and Schmid from the National College of Chiropractic near Chicago, have demonstrated a decrease in prostaglandin levels after chiropractic manipulation in women with primary dysmenorrhea.[68] This appears to be a reason for clinical success with such patients. Again, here is another field requiring further research to determine why some sub-groups of patients achieve excellent results and other do not.

D. Preventive Care and Health Promotion

As is clear from Chapter 5, "Principles and Goals of Chiropractic Practice" and the above section, preventive care and health promotion represent a large part of chiropractic education and practice. Chiropractic clinical guidelines devote chapters to the subject,[69,70] and there are texts such as *Health Promotion for Chiropractic Practice* by Jamison.[71] The role of chiropractors in this field may be summarized with examples as follows:

1. **General Clinical Practice**

   a) *Prevention/Health Promotion Similar to Medical Practice*, This includes:

   - Preventive and rehabilitative exercises to improve muscle flexibility, strength and endurance and general cardiovascular fitness to prevent fu-

ture musculoskeletal pain and disability. Three books published by chiropractors during the past year are *The Active Health and Fitness Book*,[72] *The Back Tracks Program: Your Complete Guide to Spinal Flexibility, Strength and Stability*,[73] and *Stretching for Fitness, Health and Performance: The Complete Handbook for all Ages and Fitness Levels*.[74]

   - Postural education and advice.

   - Advice on other aspects of a healthy lifestyle including nutrition, general activities of daily living and ergonomics (work space design, habits, and postures).

   b) *Chiropractic Prevention/Health Promotion*. Periodic reassessment of the neuro-musculoskeletal system, adjustment/manipulation to remove spinal subluxation/dysfunction, other manual therapies and therapeutic exercise with one or more of the following goals:

   - Preventing or limiting scoliosis (spinal curvature) and other postural distortions.

   - Improving general health by allowing the body's self-healing capacity to function normally. (See discussions on holism, homeostasis and the regu-

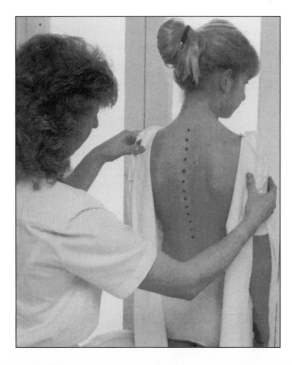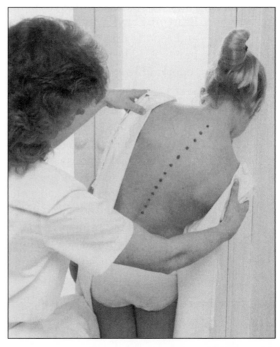

Scoliosis check up in children. Signs of scoliosis (spinal curvature) can develop early in life and all children should be checked for such signs. When caught early, most scoliosis can be halted or helped with chiropractic treatment. More severe cases, however, will still need surgery.

latory role of the nervous system in Chapter 5, "Principles and Goals of Chiropractic Care".)

- Preventing pain and disability before it arises. For example many patients with recurring mechanical joint problems, because of lifestyle, past trauma and degenerative wear and tear, have their problems successfully managed rather than cured under chiropractic care. The bus driver sitting and pulling on the wheel, the nurse bathing patients, the secretary at the computer, the professional violinist playing for hours daily, can feel increasing joint and muscular tension. They discover that certain exercises and lifestyle modifications are not sufficient alone to prevent recurring episodes of acute pain and disability, but are in combination with a chiropractic assessment and adjustment every 4–6 weeks.

The same applies to many patients with arthritis. Many people suffer significant limitations in daily activities due to arthritis. Some choose to have preventive/supportive chiropractic care enabling them to maintain functional status without heavy reliance upon medication.

2. **Specialized Activities**

a) *Individual Consulting Work.* Many chiropractors, including those with postgraduate chiropractic qualifications in the specialties of occupational health, rehabilitation and sports sciences, act as consultants in the field of education, industry, entertainment and sports.

In the U.S. Dr. Scott Donkin, author of *Sitting on the Job,*[75] is a consultant to U.S. Airways on airline seating, and Dr. Alan Powell has a similar role with Ansett Airways in Australia. Dr. Murray Miller and Dr. Lyman Johnson of Canada have respectively designed a backstrap used by mail carriers throughout North America to better support their lower backs while carrying loads, and a pelvic *Powerbelt* used by many thousands of prospective mothers and others to avoid postural strain and disability by stabilizing a progressively loosening pelvis.

Donkin's *BACKSAFE* and *SITTINGSAFE* employee training programs for the prevention of neck and back injuries are now in wide use with major corporations because of impressive results such as:

- United Airlines, after training 20,000 flight attendants in 10 countries with the *Backsafe* program led by chiropractors as trainers, saw a 63% decrease in neck and back injuries.[76,77]

- At Boeing there was a 41% reduction in back injuries.[77]

- Citicorp in Beverly Hills experienced a 50% reduction in back injuries after employees received *Sittingsafe* training. Similar results with corporations such as Chevron and Merrill Lynch have led to national contracts for employee training.[77]

b) *Professional Association Programs.* These include the design and endorsement of sleeping products in many countries. A Canadian Chiropractic Association Spinal Health Week program for elementary school children has *Inspector Spine* looking for good and bad posture, the right and wrong ways to sit at the desk or carry books, and activities that are likely to lead to playground injuries. The Chiropractors' Association of Australia has *Spinosaurus* serving a similar role in school spinal health programs.

E. **Duration and Frequency of Care**

1. **Introduction**. What is an appropriate number and frequency of treatments for a patient with acute, uncomplicated low-back pain, another with chronic headaches, and a third wanting preventive care? These are obviously important questions for everyone:

- patients, who need to assess the cost, results and when they can reasonably expect to return to normal activities;

- employers and other third party payers who are very interested in the same things;

- family physicians and others referring patients for a course of chiropractic treatment; and

- chiropractors themselves as their clinical research community better defines appropriateness of care and as they engage in contract negotiations with chiropractic networks and other managed care organizations.

At one end of the scale there are horror stories of patients consulting a chiropractor who says that 100 treatments will be necessary to solve the complex problems of their spines, and that they can open lump sum trust accounts at the office to cover payment. If this happens, refuse treatment, warn your friends and then call the state regulatory board. At the other end of the scale there are HMOs and other managed care organizations that seek to limit treatments to 3 to 6 chiropractic visits. All authorities on manipulation and spinal rehabilitation accept that this is inadequate for most patients. So, how frequently and for how long should you expect to receive treatment?

2. **Chiropractic Clinical Guidelines**. Frequency and duration of care are issues on which the chiropractic profession has established formal clinical guidelines.[76,77] The guidelines in the U.S. and Canada are, as one would expect, very similar and are summarized in the treatment charts or algorithms that appear on the following three pages. These algorithms should be clear upon careful reading, but additional summary comments are:

a) *Acute Uncomplicated Pain (Algorithm 1)*

- This algorithm applies to patients with acute pain for 3 weeks or less. It provides for 3–5 treatments a week for 4 weeks. If there is no documented improvement within 2 weeks treatment should be modified or the patient referred for other care.

    If there is modified care but still no documented improvement at 4 weeks treatment should stop with the patient referred to another professional for a second opinion.

- Typically such a patient is treated up to 3 times weekly for 2 weeks, then 3 times to 1 time weekly in the next 2 weeks depending upon progress, reinjury, etc. This amounts to 8–12 treatments over 4 weeks.

- If there is documented improvement (e.g. in terms of patient disability questionnaires, pain scales, objective measures of range of motion and pressure tenderness, etc., recorded in the patient's file) treatment may continue for up to another 4 weeks, or 8 weeks total.

U.S. and Canadian Chiropractic Clinical Guidelines.

Guidelines for Chiropractic Quality Assurance and Practice Parameters

Proceedings of the Mercy Center Consensus Conference

Edited by

Scott Haldeman, DC, MD, PhD
Commission Chairman

David Chapman-Smith, LLB
Commission Counsel

Donald M. Petersen, Jr., BS
Commission Secretary

AN ASPEN PUBLICATION®
Aspen Publishers, Inc.
Gaithersburg, Maryland
1993

CLINICAL GUIDELINES FOR CHIROPRACTIC PRACTICE IN CANADA

*Proceedings of a Consensus Conference
Commissioned by the Canadian Chiropractic Association
Held at the Glenerin Inn
Mississauga, Ontario, Canada
April 3-7, 1993.*

Edited by:

Donald Henderson, BSc, DC, FCCS(C), FCCR(C)
Chair, CCA Practice Guidelines Committee

David Chapman-Smith, LLB
Commission Counsel

Silvano Mior DC, FCCS(C)
CCA Practice Guidelines Committee

Howard Vernon, DC, FCCS(C)
CCA Practice Guidelines Committee

Algorithm 1
Based upon The Canadian Chiropractic Association Guidelines (Glenerin, 1993)

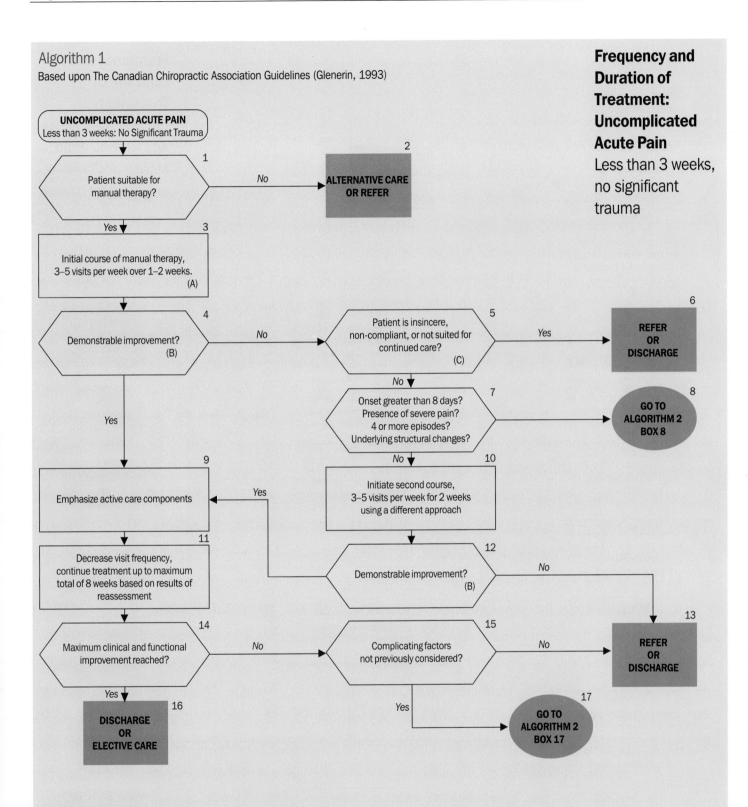

Frequency and Duration of Treatment: Uncomplicated Acute Pain
Less than 3 weeks, no significant trauma

UNCOMPLICATED ACUTE PAIN
Less than 3 weeks: No Significant Trauma

1. Patient suitable for manual therapy?
   - No → 2. ALTERNATIVE CARE OR REFER
   - Yes →
3. Initial course of manual therapy, 3–5 visits per week over 1–2 weeks. (A)
4. Demonstrable improvement? (B)
   - No → 5. Patient is insincere, non-compliant, or not suited for continued care? (C)
     - Yes → 6. REFER OR DISCHARGE
     - No → 7. Onset greater than 8 days? Presence of severe pain? 4 or more episodes? Underlying structural changes?
       - → 8. GO TO ALGORITHM 2 BOX 8
       - No → 10. Initiate second course, 3–5 visits per week for 2 weeks using a different approach
   - Yes → 9. Emphasize active care components
10. → 12. Demonstrable improvement? (B)
    - Yes → 9. Emphasize active care components
    - No → 13. REFER OR DISCHARGE
9. Emphasize active care components → 11. Decrease visit frequency, continue treatment up to maximum total of 8 weeks based on results of reassessment → 14. Maximum clinical and functional improvement reached?
    - No → 15. Complicating factors not previously considered?
      - No → 13. REFER OR DISCHARGE
      - Yes → 17. GO TO ALGORITHM 2 BOX 17
    - Yes → 16. DISCHARGE OR ELECTIVE CARE

Annotation A: Promotion of active care and the prescription of exercises should be initiated as soon as possible.
Annotation B: Improvement measured objectively, e.g., Oswestry Back Pain Disability Index, Neck Disability Index, pain scales, physiological measurements such as range of motion or muscle strength.
Annotation C: Patients may present with underlying conditions that make spinal manual therapy inappropriate or that require psychological assessment.

© Courtesy of Ontario Chiropractic Association, ©1996

Algorithm 2
Based upon The Canadian Chiropractic Association Guidelines (Glenerin, 1993)

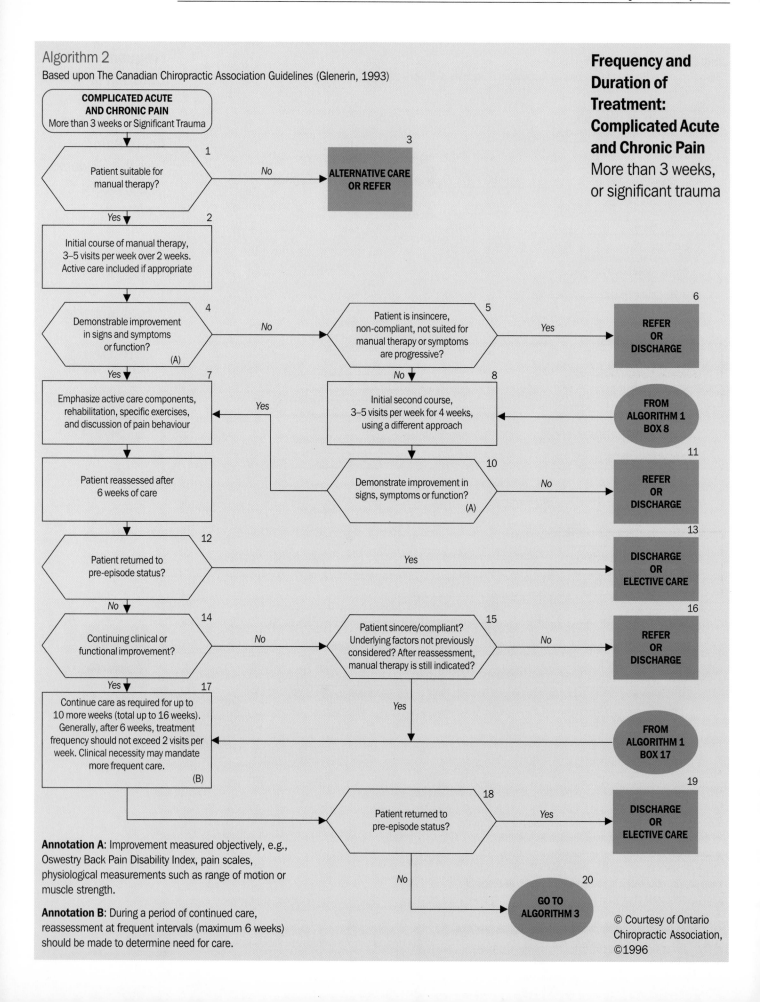

COMPLICATED ACUTE AND CHRONIC PAIN
More than 3 weeks or Significant Trauma

1 Patient suitable for manual therapy?

No → 3 **ALTERNATIVE CARE OR REFER**

Yes ↓

2 Initial course of manual therapy, 3–5 visits per week over 2 weeks. Active care included if appropriate

4 Demonstrable improvement in signs and symptoms or function? (A)

No → 5 Patient is insincere, non-compliant, not suited for manual therapy or symptoms are progressive?

Yes → 6 **REFER OR DISCHARGE**

No ↓

8 Initial second course, 3–5 visits per week for 4 weeks, using a different approach

← **FROM ALGORITHM 1 BOX 8**

Yes (to box 7)

7 Emphasize active care components, rehabilitation, specific exercises, and discussion of pain behaviour

10 Demonstrate improvement in signs, symptoms or function? (A)

No → 11 **REFER OR DISCHARGE**

Patient reassessed after 6 weeks of care

12 Patient returned to pre-episode status?

Yes → 13 **DISCHARGE OR ELECTIVE CARE**

No ↓

14 Continuing clinical or functional improvement?

No → 15 Patient sincere/compliant? Underlying factors not previously considered? After reassessment, manual therapy is still indicated?

No → 16 **REFER OR DISCHARGE**

Yes ↓

17 Continue care as required for up to 10 more weeks (total up to 16 weeks). Generally, after 6 weeks, treatment frequency should not exceed 2 visits per week. Clinical necessity may mandate more frequent care. (B)

← **FROM ALGORITHM 1 BOX 17**

18 Patient returned to pre-episode status?

Yes → 19 **DISCHARGE OR ELECTIVE CARE**

No ↓

20 **GO TO ALGORITHM 3**

Annotation A: Improvement measured objectively, e.g., Oswestry Back Pain Disability Index, pain scales, physiological measurements such as range of motion or muscle strength.

Annotation B: During a period of continued care, reassessment at frequent intervals (maximum 6 weeks) should be made to determine need for care.

© Courtesy of Ontario Chiropractic Association, ©1996

Algorithm 3
Based upon The Canadian Chiropractic Association Guidelines (Glenerin, 1993)

Frequency and Duration of Treatment: Supportive Care
After Acute or Chronic Pain Treatment has Ended

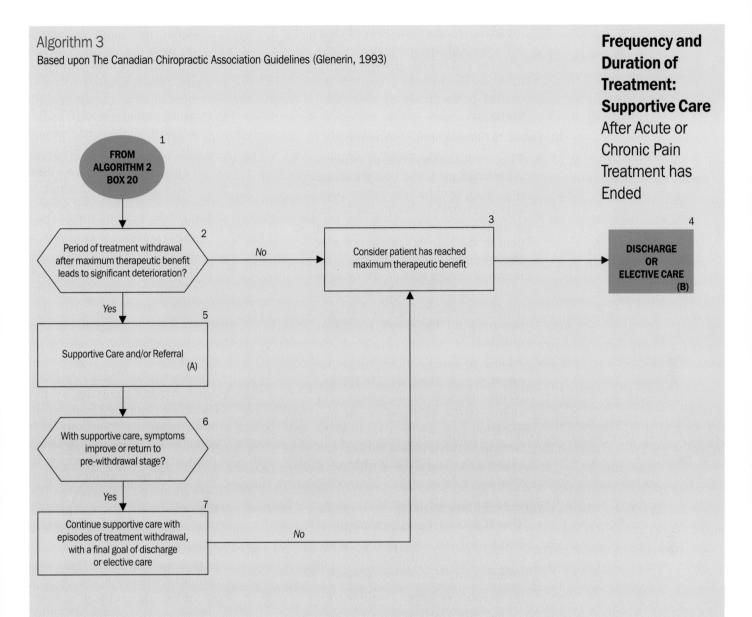

1

FROM ALGORITHM 2 BOX 20

2

Period of treatment withdrawal after maximum therapeutic benefit leads to significant deterioration?

No →

3

Consider patient has reached maximum therapeutic benefit

4

DISCHARGE OR ELECTIVE CARE (B)

Yes

5

Supportive Care and/or Referral (A)

6

With supportive care, symptoms improve or return to pre-withdrawal stage?

Yes

7

Continue supportive care with episodes of treatment withdrawal, with a final goal of discharge or elective care

No

Annotation A: Supportive care is therapeutically necessary care for patients who, despite rehabilitative exercises and other lifestyle modifications, fail to sustain therapeutic gains after treatment withdrawal. Reasons may include the ongoing stresses of work and other activities of daily living.

Annotation B: Elective care/treatment is at the option of the patient who wishes to maintain optimum function with preventive/maintenance care. Some patients, for example, wish to have functional pathology treated before pain and disability develop.

- Frequency of care drops to 1 or 2 visits per week. The frequency chosen may relate to various factors—including, for example, the need to monitor the correct performance of prescribed exercises.

b) *Pain with Complications (Algorithm 2)*

- This algorithm applies to patients with acute pain and complications (e.g. significant trauma, severe pain, significant underlying spinal degeneration, a disc problem with referred pain to the leg, etc) or recurring or chronic pain (e.g. this is the most recent of several disabling attacks of spinal pain, or the back pain/shoulder pain/headache/leg pain has been experienced for many weeks or months).

- Treatment may be slightly more frequent (e.g. 3 times weekly for 4–6 weeks, then 2 times weekly for another 4–6 weeks) and for a longer duration (e.g. up to a total of 16 weeks). However, many patients can expect a successful result within 4–6 weeks.

c) *Supportive Care (Algorithm 3)*

- The U.S. and Canadian national guidelines for chiropractic practice[69,70] define two different forms of longer term chiropractic treatment:

  i) ***Supportive care***. Treatment for patients who have reached maximum improvement, but who fail to sustain this improvement and progressively deteriorate when treatment is withdrawn. (In other words, *supportive care* is necessary from the patient's point of view.)

  ii) ***Preventive/Maintenance Care***. Treatment for a patient who has no present pain or symptoms but seeks to prevent pain and disability, promote health and enhance the quality of life. (In other words, *preventive/maintenance care* is not therapeutically necessary from the patient's point of view, but is optional or elective.)

    - Algorithm 3 illustrates the role of supportive care. It does not explain how many treatments are involved because, as the U.S. and Canadian guidelines say, "the frequency of treatment must be determined on an individual case basis as dictated by therapeutic necessity."

    - Typically supportive care might involve 3–6 treatments over 2 weeks to arrest returning pain and disability, then one treatment every 2–4 weeks for a settling period of a few months and then another attempt at complete withdrawal of care.

Rarely there will be patients who require supportive care on an almost weekly basis. The case of *Lynch v Halifax Insurance Company*, a 1994 decision by the Ontario Insurance Commission in Canada,[78] is an example. It accepted the distinction between supportive care, necessary to maintain improvement and prevent disability following earlier injury and treatment, and preventive/maintenance care, which is elective.

In this case Mr. Lynch, who sustained a whiplash injury in a motor vehicle accident in 1990, was receiving continuing chiropractic care four years later. Halifax, his insurer, refused to pay for the continuing care and claimed it was an "unending series of treatments" that was passive, created patient dependency and was not necessary or reasonable. Mr. Lynch disputed this, saying his continuing chiropractic care was both reasonable and necessary because it maintained his ability to stay at work and perform his normal activities of daily living. The continuing use of chiropractic treatments was just as reasonable as the continuing use of drugs to control a chronic recurring pain problem.

The arbitrator agreed with Mr. Lynch. On the facts of the case, which included the particular demands of Mr. Lynch's job, and the evidence that he kept himself physically fit and was well motivated but needed some ongoing care to avoid deterioration and disability, the arbitrator ruled that the ongoing care was supportive care, not preventative/maintenance care, and that the insurer was liable for payment.

d) *Preventive Care*

- This has been defined in the above section on supportive care. It is elective—some patients concerned with the early detection and correction of neuromusculoskeletal disorders will choose preventive/maintenance care, others will not.

- Frequency of preventive care depends upon a number of factors including the patient's lifestyle, work habits and general health. Many patients have a preventive care visit every 3 or 6 months.

3. **Clinical Trials.** How many treatment visits have been used in clinical trials studying the effectiveness of chiropractic care? This varies according to the condition.

- For patients with chronic back pain, neck pain and headache there are typically 10-20 treatments over 6 weeks to 3 months.

  In Boline et al.'s trial showing successful chiropractic management of chronic tension-type headache, patients received treatment and advice 2 times weekly for 6 weeks.[22] In another tension-type headache trial now underway in Canada patients are receiving treatment and advice 3 times weekly for 6 weeks.[79] For chronic back pain Kirkaldy-Willis and Cassidy provided up to 15 treatments,[80] and Bronfort et al. 20 treatments (manipulation and exercise 2 times weekly for 5 weeks, then 10 exercise sessions over the next 6 weeks).[81] Meade et al., who mixed acute and chronic patients, provided only 10 treatments but over 3 months.[82]

- In a recent trial for adolescent patients

with asthma there was greater frequency and duration. Patients received chiropractic treatment 3 times weekly for 4 weeks, then 2 times weekly for 4 weeks, then once weekly for 8 weeks, comprising a total of 28 visits over 16 weeks. (Some variation was allowed—patients were to receive between 20-36 treatments over a period of up to 4 months).[40]

- For a study of chiropractic management of infantile colic, a condition with a high natural remission rate, the duration and frequency of care were much less. Infants received up to 3 treatments over 2 weeks.[44]

In summary, the clinical trials give some guidance on frequency and duration of care but no clear direction. One reason is that the budgets for trials often provide artificial limitations of time and cost. Another is that, as yet, there is simply insufficient study of the required number of visits for optimum results for most patients with various given conditions. The national U.S. and Canadian guidelines referred to in paragraph 2, which combine the information from published studies and clinical experience, provide the best possible information at present.

4. **Third Party Coverage/Managed Care**. Many factors affect the level of third party and managed care coverage of chiropractic services, which varies tremendously, so this gives little guidance on what amounts to a reasonable course of chiropractic care. In the province of Ontario, Canada, where chiropractic services are fully integrated into the health care system:

- The provincial government's health care plan provides coverage for up to 22 visits per person per year for chiropractic services.

- Auto insurance law provides mandatory coverage of "reasonable and necessary" chiropractic services after an accident. There is automatic entitlement to 16 visits in the first 8 weeks post-accident for all health care professionals including chiropractors, then coverage pursuant to a treatment plan filed with the insurer. For Grade 2 and 3 whiplash injuries (essentially documented neck strains and sprains) a treatment plan providing for care up to 3 months in accordance with the frequency given above in the chiropractic guidelines will be viewed as reasonable and necessary.

- Workers' compensation provides that an injured worker may choose chiropractic care, which can be given as deemed appropriate for 12 weeks, but thereafter only on approval from the Board. Extensions after 12 weeks are often not necessary, but when sought are given if there is proper cause shown on the file.

5. **Real and Unreal Guidelines**. Clinical guidelines, giving directions on best current practice of a profession, are developed not only for the profession but also the public. There is a formal and recognized process for developing them, involving review of the evidence by a properly representative group in the profession. This process was followed for the U.S. and Canadian guidelines referred to in this section.

In 1998 another chiropractic clinical guideline was distributed in the U.S. by the impressive sounding Council on Chiropractic Practice. This is a small splinter group not representative of the profession. With respect to duration and frequency of care, its guideline titled *Vertebral Subluxation in Chiropractic Practice*[83] provides a basis for unlimited chiropractic treatments. The chapter on duration of care provides no numbers or time frames and puts no limits on the judgement of the individual chiropractor. Readers should know that this guideline does not follow accepted rules of evidence (as explained in Section C, Chapter 1) and has been rejected by all major organizations in the chiropractic profession.

6. **Conclusion**. It is important to remember that the natural history for many chiropractic patients, meaning the expected improvement rate even without treatment by anyone, is that their soft-tissue injuries and pain will resolve within 6 weeks. Under effective care these patients should improve considerably more quickly than that.

The above discussion represents an overview covering a very wide range of patients. Some will require only one or a few treatments, others with multiple injuries and complications may be receiving daily treatment for several months in a chiropractic rehabilitation facility.

References

1　Yochum TR, Rowe LJ. Essentials of skeletal radiology. Baltimore, Maryland: Williams and Wilkins, 1987.

2　Marchiori DM. Clinical imaging: with skeletal chest and abdomen pattern differentials. St Louis, Missouri: Mosby Yearbook, 1999.

3　Christensen M, Morgan D, eds. Job analysis of chiropractic: a project report, survey analysis and summary of the practice of chiropractic within the United States. Greely, Colorado: National Board of Chiropractic Examiners, 1993.

4　Hurwitz EL, Coulter ID, et al. Use of chiropractic services from 1985 through 1991 in the United States and Canada. 1990-1997. JAMA 1998;280:1569–75.

5　Bergmann TF, Peterson DH, Lawrence DL. Chiropractic technique. New York: Churchill Livingstone, 1993.

6　Liebenson C, ed. Rehabilitation of the spine: A practitioner's manual. Baltimore, Maryland: Williams and Wilkins, 1996.

7　Hochschuler S, ed. Rehabilitation of the spine. St. Louis, Missouri: Mosby, 1993.

8　Sherwood P. Effective prevention of coronary heart attacks. Digest Chiro Econ 1985;54–7,122–3. (Reprinted from Am J Acupunct 1984.)

9　Nicholas AS, DeBias DA, et al. A somatic component to myocardial infarction. Br Med J 1985;291:13–7.

10　Lord SM, Barnsley L, et al. Chronic cervical zygapophysial joint pain after whiplash. A placebo-controlled prevalence study. Spine 1996;21:1737–45.

11　Hack GD, Koritzer RT, et al. Anatomic relation between the rectus capitis posterior minor muscle and the dura mater. Spine 1995;20:2484–6.

12　Mitchell BS, Humphreys BK, Sullivan E. Attachments of the ligamentum nuchae to cervical posterior spinal dura and the lateral part of the occipital bone. J Manip Physiol Ther 1998;21:145–8.

13　Spitzer WO, Skovron ML, et al. Scientific monograph of the Quebec task force on whiplash-associated disorders: redefining whiplash and its management. Spine 1995;20:8S.

14　Coulter ID, Hurwitz EL, et al. The appropriateness of manipulation and mobilization of the cervical spine. Santa Monica, California: RAND, 1996; Document No. MR-781-CR.

15　Hurwitz El, Aker PD, Adams AH, Meeker WC, Shekelle PG. Manipulation and mobilization of the cervical spine: a systematic review of the literature. Spine 1996;21:1746–60.

16　Cassidy JD. Expert evidence at the Mathiason Inquest. Coroner's Court, Saskatoon, Saskatchewan, Canada. 1998: Transcript 873–875.

17　Aker PD, Gross AR, et al. Conservative management of mechanical neck pain: systematic overview and meta-analysis. Br Med J 1996;313:1291–96.

18　Haldeman S, Kohlbeck FJ, McGregor M. Risk Factors and Precipitating Neck Movements Causing Vertebrobasilar Artery Dissection After Cervical Trauma and Spinal Manipulation, Spine 1999;24(8):785–794.

19　Parker G, Tupling H, Pryor D. A controlled trial of cervical manipulation for migraine. Aust NZ J Med 1978;8:589–93.

20 Parker GB, et al. Why does migraine improve during a clinical trial? Further results from a trial of cervical manipulation for migraine. Aust NZ J Med 1980;10:192–8.

21 Nelson CF, Bronfort G, et al. The efficacy of spinal manipulation, amitriptyline and the combination of both therapies for the prophylaxis of migraine headache. J Manip Physiol Ther 1998;21:511–9.

22 Boline P, Kassak K, Bronfort G, Nelson C, Anderson A. Spinal manipulation vs amitriptyline for the treatment of chronic tension-type headaches. J Manip Physiol Ther 1995;18:148–54.

23 Nilsson N, Christensen HW, et al. The effect of spinal manipulation in the treatment of cervicogenic headache. J Manip Physiol Ther 1997;20:326–30.

24 Tuchin PJ, Pollard H, Bonello R. A Randomized Controlled Trial of Chiropractic Spinal Manipulation Therapy for Migraine. Proceedings of the 5th Biennial Congress of the World Federation of Chiropractic, 1999:183–184, Abstract. In print.

25 Sjaastad O, et al. Cervicogenic headache, C_2 rhizopathy, and occipital neuralgia: a connection. Cephalalgia 1986;6:189–95,194.

26 Saper JR. Migraine, migraine variance and related vascular headaches. In: Jacobson AC, Donlon WC, eds. Headache and facial pain: diagnosis and management. New York: Raven Press, 1990; 81–82.

27 Nilsson N. The prevalence of cervicogenic headache in a random population sample of 20-50 year-olds. Spine 1995;20:1884–8.

28 Curl DD. Chiropractic approach to head pain. Baltimore, Maryland: Williams and Wilkins, 1994.

29 Steigerwald DP, Croft AC, et al. Whiplash and temporomandibular disorders. An interdisciplinary approach to case management. San Diego, California: Keiser Publishing, 1992.

30 Davis PT, Hulbert JR, et al. Comparative efficacy of conservative medical and chiropractic treatments for carpal tunnel syndrome: a randomized clinical trial. J Manip Physiol Ther 1998;21:317–26.

31 Bonebrake AR, Fernandez JE, et al. A treatment for carpal tunnel syndrome: results of a follow-up study. J Manip Physiol Ther 1993;16:125–9.

32 Sucher BM. Palpatory diagnosis and manipulative management of carpal tunnel syndrome. JAOA 1994;94:647-63.

33 Winters JC, Sobel JS, et al. Comparison of physiotherapy, manipulation, and corticosteroid injection for treating shoulder complaints in general practice: randomized, single blind study. Br Med J 1993;314:1320–5.

34 Suter, E McMorland G et al. Effects of Sacroiliac Joint Manipulation on Quadriceps Inhibition in Patients with Anterior Knee Pain: A Randomized Controlled Trial. Proceedings of the 5th Biennial Congress of the World Federation of Chiropractic, 1999:181–182, Abstract. In print.

35 Mennell J. Joint pain: diagnosis and treatment using manipulative techniques. Boston, Massachusetts: Little, Brown, 1964.

36 Stoddard A. Manual of osteopathic practice. 2nd edition. London, England: Hutchinson & Co, 1983.

37 Hasselberg PD. Chiropractic in New Zealand. Report of Commission of Inquiry into Chiropractic. Wellington, New Zealand: Government Printer, 1979.

38 Ref 37 supra, Chapter 32.

39 Hviid C. A comparison of the effect of chiropractic treatment on respiratory function in patients with respiratory distress symptoms and patients without. Bull Eur Chiro Union 1978;26:17–34.

40 Balon J, Aker PD, Crowther ER, et al. A comparison of active and simulated chiropractic manipulation as adjunctive treatment for childhood asthma. NEJM 1998;339:1013–20.

41 Brønfort G. Asthma and chiropractic. Eur J Chiro 1996;44:1–7.

42 LeBoeuf-Yde C, Brown P, et al. Chiropractic care of children with nocturnal enuresis: a prospective outcome study. J Manip Physiol Ther 1991;14:110–5.

43 Reed WR, Beavers S, Reddy SK, Kern G. Chiropractic management of primary nocturnal enuresis. J Manip Physiol Ther 1994;17(9):596–600.

44 Klougart N, Nilsson N, Jacobsen J. Infantile colic treated by chiropractors: a prospective study of 316 Cases.

J Manip Physiol Ther 1989;12:281–8.

45 Gutmann G. The atlas fixation syndrome in the baby and infant. Manuelle Medizin 1987;25:5–10, Trans. Peters RE.

46 Phillips NJ. Vertebral subluxation and otitis media: a case study, chiropractic. J Chiro Res Clin Invest 1992;8:38–9.

47 Fallon JM. The role of the chiropractic adjustment in the care and treatment of 332 children with otitis media. J J Clin Chiro Ped 1997;2:167–83.

48 Froehle RM. Ear infection: a retrospective study examining improvement from chiropractic care and analyzing for influencing factors. J Manip Physiol Ther 1996;19:169–77.

49 Lewit K. Manipulative therapy and rehabilitation of the locomotor system. 2nd ed. Oxford, England: Butterworth-Heineman, 1991:273.

50 Bourdillon JF. Spinal manipulation. 3rd ed. London, England: William Heinemann Medical Books, 1982: 6, 205–206, 218–219.

51 Gilman G, Bergstrand J. Visual recovery following chiropractic intervention. J Behavioral Optometry 1(3). Reprinted in California Chiropractic Journal 1990:15:22–8.

52 Gorman RF. Monocular visual loss after closed head trauma: immediate resolution associated with spinal manipulation. J Manip Physiol Ther 1995;18:308–14.

53 Stephens D, Mealing D, et al. Treatment of visual field loss by spinal manipulation: a report on 17 patients. JNMS 1998;6:53–66.

54 Fitz-Ritson D. Assessment of cervicogenic vertigo. J Manip Physiol Ther 1991;14:193–8.

55 Bracher E, Bleggi C, Almeida C et al. A Combined Approach for The Treatment of Cervical Vertigo. Proceedings of the 5th Biennial Congress of the World Federation of Chiropractic, 1999:154–155. In print.

56 Ref 49 supra, 327, 329.

57 Yates RG, Lamping DL, et al. Effects of chiropractic treatment on blood pressure and anxiety: a randomized, controlled trial. J Manip Physiol Ther 1998;11:484–8.

58 Ref 37 supra, 164.

59 Miller WD. Treatment of visceral disorders by manipulative therapy. In: Goldstein M. The research status of spinal manipulative therapy. Bethesda, Maryland: NINCDS Monograph, U.S. Department of Health, Education and Welfare, 1975:295–301.

60 Bronfort G, Evans R, et al. Is chiropractic spinal manipulation an effective co-management strategy for pediatric asthma? Results of a prospective case series and pilot study. Montreal, Quebec: North American Primary Care Research Group, November 5–8, 1998. In print.

61 Lewit K. Ein fall von auftahrunfall. Manuelle Medizin 1975:13:71.

62 Rychlikova E. Schmerzen im gallonblazan bereich auf grund vertebragener storungen. Deutsches Gesundheitswesen 1975:29,2092.

63 Pikalov AA, Vyatcheslav VK. Use of spinal manipulative therapy in the treatment of duodenal ulcer: a pilot study. J Manip Physiol Ther 1994;17:310–3.

64 Kunert W. Functional disorders of internal organs due to vertebral lesions. CIBA Symposium. Bonn: University Medical Polyclinic, 1965:13(3).

65 Sato A, Swenson RS. Sympathetic nervous system response to mechanical stress of the spinal column in rats. J Manip Physiol Ther 1984;7:141–7.

66 Budgell B, Hotta H, Sato A. Spinovisceral reflexes evoked by noxious and innocuous stimulation of the lumbar spine. JNMS 1995;3:122–31.

67 Browning JE. Chiropractic distractive decompression in the treatment of pelvic pain and organic dysfunction in patients with evidence of lower sacral nerve root compression. J Manip Phyisol Ther 1988;11:436–42.

68 Kokjohn K, Schmid DC, et al. The effect of spinal manipulation on pain and prostaglandin levels in women with primary dysmenorrhea. J Manip Physiol Ther 1992;15:279–85.

69 Haldeman S, Chapman-Smith D, Petersen DM, eds. Guidelines for chiropractic quality assurance and practice parameters. Gaithersburg, Maryland: Aspen Publishers, 1992.

70 Henderson DJ, et al, eds. Clinical guidelines for chiropractic practice in Canada. Suppl. to JCCA 1994;38(1).

71 Jamison JR. The chiropractic as health information resource; health promotion for chiropractic practice. Gaithersburg, Maryland: Aspen Publishers, 1991.

72 Jongsma DM. The active health and fitness book. Ontario, Canada: Barrie Press, 1998.

73 Panetta L. The backtracks program: your complete guide to spinal flexibility, strength and stability, DocuLink International, 1999.

74 Oswald CA, Bacso SN. Stretching for fitness, health and performance: the complete handbook for all ages and fitness levels. New York: Sterling Publishing Company, 1998.

75 Donkin SW. Sitting on the job: a practical survival guide for people who earn their living while sitting. Lincoln, Nebraska: Parallel Integration, 1987.

76 Bigos S, Bowyer O, Braen G, et al. Acute low-back problems in adults. Clinical practice guideline No.14. Rockville, Maryland: Agency for Health Care Policy and Research, Public Health Service, U.S. Department of Health and Human Services, 1994; AHCPR Publication No. 95-0642.

77 Rosen M, Breen A, et al. Management guidelines for back pain. Appendix B in Report of a clinical standards advisory group committee on back pain. London, England: Her Majesty's Stationery Office (HMSO), 1994.

78 Lynch v The Halifax Insurance Company, OIC File No. A-004781, Decision dated December 20, 1994). Note: For guidelines on preventative/maintenance care see Chapter 14 of the CCA Guidelines.

79 Vernon H, Jansz G et al. 1999. Trial Proposal.

80 Kirkaldy-Willis WH, Cassidy JD. Spinal manipulation in the treatment of low-back pain. Can Fam Phys 1985;31:535–40.

81 Bronfort G, Goldsmith CH, et al. Trunk exercise with spinal manipulative or NSAID therapy for chronic low-back pain: a randomized, observer-blinded clinical trial. J Manip Physiol Ther 1986;19:576–83.

82 Meade TW, Dyer S, et al. Low-back pain of mechanical origin: randomised comparison of chiropractic and hospital outpatient treatment. Br Med J 1990;300:1431–7.

83 Vertebral subluxation in chiropractic practice. Chandler, Arizona: Council on Chiropractic Practice, 1998.

CHAPTER 7

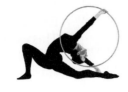

MANIPULATION

A. Definition

The terms "spinal manipulation" and "spinal manipulative therapy" are often used by lay persons and professionals to refer to all manual techniques used to treat muscles or joints. During the past fifteen years the following definitions have become distinct in the international health science literature with respect to treatment of joint disorders:

Mobilization. Slower or low-velocity techniques in which the joint remains within its passive range of movement. The treatment can be monitored and resisted by the patient, who therefore has final control.

Manipulation. Faster or high-velocity techniques that take the joint beyond the passive range end barrier to what is known as the paraphysiological space. Range of movement is greater. Because of the speed, the patient does not have control. Potential for harm in unskilled hands is greater.

Another way of explaining the difference is that manipulation is a sudden thrust or impulse or force applied at the end of the passive range of movement that gaps the joint to a degree that cannot be achieved by mobilization. As you can see in Figure 1, which illustrates the difference between manipulation and mobilization, there are three ranges of movement in a joint:

1. **Active Range**. Turn your head to the right as far as you can. You have reached the active range end barrier of your combined neck joints.

2. **Passive Range**. Now push your left cheek with your left hand. Your neck turns further—to the passive end range barrier.

3. **Paraphysiological Range**. If you now applied angles and finger leverages to your neck but concentrated force lines at one

neck joint, and then applied a specific sudden thrust, the joint surfaces would separate—creating further motion to the paraphysiological space end barrier. However, ***do not try to do this***.

Although manipulation involves a sudden thrust with speed, it is over an extremely small range of movement—similar to the movement in the joint when you crack your fingers. It is usually accompanied by a pop or cracking sound. The technical term for this is "cavitation". This is not made by bone, but is the sound of the collapse of a bubble of gas that escapes from the joint fluid because of low pressure when the two joint surfaces are separated.

In the words of chiropractors Dr. David Cassidy and Dr. Haymo Thiel and orthopedic surgeon Dr. William Kirkaldy-Willis, leading authorities in this field, "the phenomenon of joint fluid cavitation is central to the definition and effect of manipulation." The negative pressure that normally helps to hold the cartilage joint surfaces together is temporarily decreased allowing more freedom and greater passive

Figure 1 **Manipulation and Mobilization**

Neutral

Active Range

Passive Range

Paraphysiological space

Active ROM

Mobilization

Manipulation

From Raymond Sandoz

range of motion. None of this usually occurs with mobilization. It takes approximately 20 minutes for the two joint surfaces to return to their former position and pressure.[2]

Manipulation and mobilization are terms used by all professions with an interest in manual care. The chiropractic term "adjustment," as in "joint adjustment" or "spinal adjustment," covers both types of joint treatment.

Many chiropractic techniques use speed (high-velocity), and are manipulation. Others do not (low-velocity). Some are low-velocity but still cause a pop or audible release and take the joint into the paraphysiological space. In chiropractic practice and under insurance laws these are often termed "low-velocity manipulation," but according to current scientific definitions are mobilization.

The importance of the distinction between manipulation and mobilization is underlined by the growing body of research showing that manipulation has superior results in increasing range of movement in a joint[3,4] and in treating back pain,[5] neck pain and headache.[4,6,7] Further illustration of the difference between mobilization and manipulation appears in Figure 2.

B. Professional Training

Manual diagnosis and treatment is a complex field requiring extensive full-time education. This exists at the undergraduate or first professional level in chiropractic, and in osteopathy in Australia and the U.K. It is also found at the postgraduate level for osteopathy in the U.S., and for physical therapy in Australia and several European countries. Leaders in all relevant professions, including medical specialists with experience of manual medicine, agree that weekend and part-time courses are inadequate.

The only government commission that has looked at this issue thoroughly, in New Zealand, concluded that "part-time or vacation courses for health professionals should not be encouraged" and that medical doctors would require 12 months full-time training "to acquire a degree of diagnostic and manual skill sufficient to match chiropractic standards." Physical therapists would require longer training than that.[8]

This is a problem area. In the past 15 years spinal joint manipulation and mobilization, now firmly established as part of the first line of treatment for most patients with back pain and neck pain, have become increasingly popular.

Figure 2 **Ranges of Joint Motion During Active Movement, Mobilization and Manipulation.**

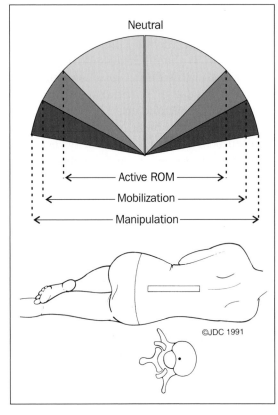

Figure 2.1 **The spine and joint at rest.**

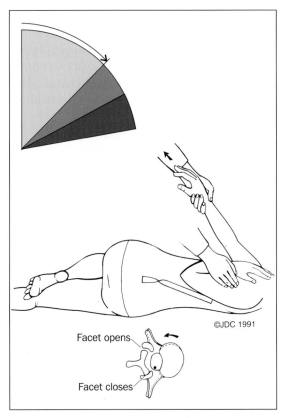

Figure 2.2 **Active movement (i.e., the movement a patient can achieve without assistance) begins to open facet joints.**

One result is increased medical referral of patients to chiropractors. Another is that informal postgraduate courses are being offered to medical doctors (MDs) and physical therapists (PTs).

The Australian Royal College of General Practitioners, through its journal *The Australian Family Physician*, offered a correspondence course.[9] In North America PT journals advertise a proliferation of weekend courses, and medical societies are teaching manipulation to MDs on the same basis and promising doctors "will then be competent to start treating patients."

What is your view of this advice to MDs in the *British Medical Journal*:[10]

"Courses including manipulation (lasting about a week) are run for doctors and physiotherapists by the Cyriax Foundation and by the Society of Orthopaedic Medicine, and intensive weekend courses for doctors are held by the British Association of Manipulative Medicine. These courses provide clinicians with the knowledge and the necessary manual skills to start treating patients safely. Doctors will then need at least six to nine months of regular practice *to begin to feel that they are treating the right patients and doing so appropriately—and years*

to become fully experienced and confident."[10] (Emphasis added.)

For a medical doctor there are three areas of specialized training required—theory (including applied anatomy, biomechanics, neurophysiology and radiology); examination and diagnosis; and treatment techniques. In U.S. osteopathy, for which the first professional program is now the equivalent of medical education, these skills are taught in a 3 year postgraduate specialty. Here are the views of leaders in manual medicine:

The great majority of doctors who learn manipulation are taught far too little about how, where, and when to use it . . . they are clinically blindfolded.

1. "The accurate appreciation of joint stiffness and, even more, that of excess tension in the muscles, requires training and . . . even with constant practice this training takes a long time. The necessity for this training is not always appreciated." John Bourdillon, MD, Canada.[11]

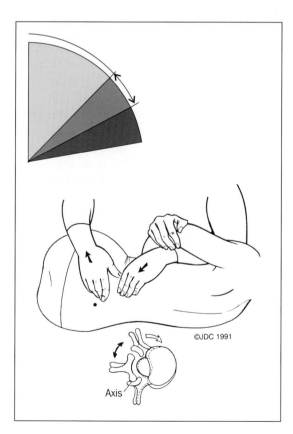

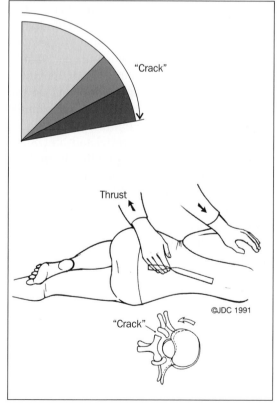

Figure 2.3 **Mobilization further increases the range of motion in the joint.**

Figure 2.4 **Manipulation increases the range of joint motion even further.**

2. "To learn when to manipulate and when not, and what sort of maneuvres to use, is a diagnostic problem involving years of study . . . (it) requires a high degree of knowledge and skill." James Cyriax, MD, England.[12]

3. "Prolonged training under guidance is indispensable." Robert Maigne, MD, France.[13]

4. "The great majority of (medical) students and doctors who learn manipulation are taught far too little about how, where, and when to use it . . . they are clinically blindfolded. The practice of spinal manipulation

There are now a number of well-described mechanical and reflex results of manipulation.

understanding all the many forms of disturbed function of the motor system requires great skill demanding long training." Karel Lewit, MD, Czech Republic.[14]

C. Full-time Practice

The Canadian orthopedic surgeon and researcher William Kirkaldy-Willis, editor of the text *Managing Low-Back Pain*,[15] advises that spinal manipulation also requires full-time practice and family physicians should refer to a chiropractor or other specialist. Alan Stoddard, DO, MD, twice qualified with respect to manipulation as an osteopath and specialist in physical medicine in England, puts it this way:

"The art of manipulation depends on the ability of the practitioner to combine the forces he uses such that the maximum leverage occurs precisely at the level of the restricted joint. Such skill takes a great deal of practice to perfect. Clearly those engaged in continuous practice are likely to be more skilled than those who manipulate only on rare occasions. The concert pianist practices his art daily to maintain a high standard. This applies equally to the art of manipulation."[16]

D. How Does Manipulation Work— Mechanisms of Action

There are now a number of well-described *mechanical* and *reflex* results of manipulation. These include:

1. Joint cavitation and increased range of motion (mechanical), causing inhibition or reduction of pain (reflex). The transmission

of pain signals up the spinal cord can be increased by lack of proprioceptive signals (sensory information to the spinal cord on the movements and positions of muscles); or reduced by greater proprioceptive input. This is Melzack and Wall's "gate" mechanism[17]—the gate is opened to pain (nociceptive signals) by reduced other sensory input.

The spinal facet joints are rich in mechanoreceptors, the nerve endings that give proprioceptive input. This is given through large nerve fibers, which compete with adjacent smaller pain fibers for central spinal cord transmission of information to the brain. Increased proprioceptive input from increased joint motion reduces—closes the gate on—pain transmission.

2. Joint and muscle receptor stimulation (mechanical) causing relaxation of paraspinal muscles (reflex). Wyke and others have shown that stimulation of the mechanoreceptors by stretching of the joint has a reflex effect on muscles over the joint, calming the muscle excitability and spasms that are often a part of low-back pain.[18]

Herzog's interdisciplinary team at the University of Calgary in Canada has recently shown that 11 commonly used chiropractic manipulative techniques for different regions of the spine and pelvis not only have calming reflex effects on muscles near the joint being manipulated but also in other areas of the spine, arms and legs. The electronogram (EMG) responses in these muscles are "clear, measurable and repeatable" and spread over a distinct and typical area.[19] (With a right-sided neck manipulation, for example, there are standard EMG responses in most muscles of the neck and back and a consistent response in the trapezius muscle in the right arm; sacroiliac joint manipulation produces consistent EMG responses in the back muscles, deltoids, and gluteal muscles.)

3. Breaking of joint adhesions (mechanical). With chronic or long-term pain there is shortening of connective tissue, long-term reduced joint mobility and formation of adhesions—the joint is partially "stuck together." Manipulation can stretch or break these adhesions. This brings increased motion which has the reflex effects already discussed.

4. Release of connective tissue trapped in joints (mechanical). Anatomical studies by Giles in Australia[20] in the 1980s showed tags of fibrous and other tissue that had become trapped in lumbar and cervical facet joints. Giles discusses how these may cause irritation and traction in both the affected joints and adjacent ones, leading to the reflex muscle spasm associated with acute locked back or neck (torticollis). Manipulation can release these tags of tissue.

5. Stimulation of the autonomic nervous system (ANS) (reflex) through cavitation and increased range of motion (mechanical). The work of Korr,[21] for example, indicates that spinal manipulation, through ANS reflex effects, influences the vasomotor tone (the caliber or diameter of blood vessels and their function) of neuromusculoskeletal tissues.

6. Relief of chronic nerve compression and irritation by correction of abnormal joint mechanics (mechanical). Joint dysfunction can directly compress or irritate nerves, especially in the canals through which spinal nerves exit from the spinal cord (interpedicular zone). While the entrance to these canals (the intervertebral foramen) is quite spacious for the exiting spinal nerve root, there is minimal spare space for the nerves and associated blood vessels in the interpedicular zone.[22] This situation is aggravated by degeneration or stenosis—narrowing of these canals because of bony outgrowths over time.

Kirkaldy-Willis and Cassidy have reported good results with many back patients with central (spinal) or lateral (nerve root canal) stenosis.[23] It is thought that many of them will have had a combination of stenosis and restricted joint motion. Manipulation increases range of motion, thereby relieving chronic intermittent nerve compression and stretch.

These views are now supported by hard research. Cohen and Triano have studied the comparative skill levels of newly trained practitioners and experienced clinicians and demonstrated clearly that, in terms of precise biomechanical performance, manipulative skills improve appreciably over time and are markedly superior in experienced professionals.[24]

E. Specific Effects of Manipulation

It was once suggested by critics of manipulation and chiropractic that, although there seemed to be results, this was only because of the "laying on of hands" and placebo or non-specific treatment effects. Manipulation might move a joint, but this did more for the mind than the body.

Chiropractic research during the 1980s showed this was wrong. Many specific effects have now been demonstrated objectively. Examples are now given. These are the proven immediate results of a single chiropractic

Many specific effects [of manipulation] have now been demonstrated objectively.

adjustment or manipulation. Comment on clinical trials for treatment of various conditions, such as back pain or headache, appears in other chapters.

1. **Effects on Sensory and Motor Function.** These are effects in the musculoskeletal system, produced through mechanical changes in the central and peripheral branches of the nervous system.

   a) Increased joint range of motion in all three planes—forward/backward (anterior/ posterior); sideways (lateral); and rotation—and reduction of pain.[4,25]

   b) Increased skin pain tolerance level.[26]

   c) Increased paraspinal muscle pressure pain tolerance.[27]

   d) Reduced muscle electrical activity and tension.[28,29]

   e) Consistent, repeatable reflex responses in muscles in the spine and limbs.[19]

   With respect to b) skin pain tolerance, for example, Terrett and Vernon tested the hypothesis that local skin tolerance would increase following a single chiropractic adjustment or manipulation to a restricted joint.

   • Fifty subjects without spinal pain, but found by electrical stimulus to the skin over the T1-T10 spinal segments to have identifiable zones of increased pain, were admitted to the trial. All were found to have movement restriction in an adjacent joint or motion segment, and were told they would receive manipulation.

- Half, chosen randomly, were given one chiropractic manipulation (direct thrust/pisiform contact/to hypomobile aspect) at the level of increased pain. The other half received a joint springing maneuver as a sham or control procedure. This meant they experienced a "laying on of hands," but one with no known specific effect.

... placebo effects were the basis of treatment in former times, remain one of the most important elements of health care and should be embraced rather than rejected.

- Pain tolerance to repeat electrical stimulus was assessed at 30 seconds, 2 minutes, 5 minutes and 10 minutes. The control group had unchanged pain tolerance/sensitivity. However the group receiving a manipulation experienced a statistically significant elevation of pain tolerance (140%).

- The researchers concluded that chiropractic manipulation, as performed, increases skin pain tolerance levels. Their findings suggested "an underlying sub-clinical facilitation of cutaneous sensory reflex pathways coupled with a biomechanical fault in an adjacent motion segment."

2. **Effects on sympathetic function**. These are effects produced through the central and autonomic branches of the nervous system. The sympathetic division of the autonomic nervous system regulates visceral function, including vasomotor (blood circulation) and sudomotor (sweat gland) activity. Various studies and trials have demonstrated the immediate effect of a chiropractic adjustment or manipulation on sympathetic function including:

a) Blood flow and distal skin temperature (fingertips).[30]

b) Blood pressure.[31,32]

c) Blood chemistry. Effects include increased secretion of melatonin,[33] increased plasma beta endorphin levels,[4,34]

and elevation of substance P and enhanced neutrophil respiratory burst.[35]

d) Control of pupillary diameter.[36]

Briggs and Boone studied the effects of chiropractic adjustment on changes in pupillary diameter because this was related to a relatively well-defined autonomic pathway and was non-invasive.

Fifteen subjects, chosen following screening by an optometrist, were evaluated for four days pre-treatment to determine a baseline of pupillary diameter under controlled conditions and to establish those having cervical subluxation.

Prior to treatment subjects were dark-adapted for 15 minutes to neutralize the predominant parasympathetic control of the pupil present under normal light conditions. Pupillary diameter (PD) was then measured from sophisticated photographic studies.

Subjects with subluxation (8) were given a single manipulation (toggle recoil or modified cervical break) at the compromised level in the cervical spine—C1, C2 or C5. Those without subluxation (7) formed a control group and were given a sham adjustment comprising a slight muscle massage to the upper cervical spine. There was then repeat photographic procedures and measurement.

There were a number of interesting results. Firstly, in the 4-day pre-treatment observation period those with subluxation showed significant variations in PD day to day, whereas those without subluxation did not. Secondly, those without subluxation experienced no PD change following sham adjustment whereas those in the treatment group showed clear changes. These were variable, however, following adjustment to C2 and C5 there was a sympathetic response (dilation), following adjustment of C1 a parasympathetic response (constriction).

The investigators concluded that subluxation and adjustment effect a response in PD mediated by the autonomic nervous system. They suggest that "the observed autonomic responses seen in this investigation ... may be reflections of neural summation of segmental afferent and supra-spinal descend ing fibers on sympathetic pre-ganglionic neurons."[36]

F. Non-Specific or Placebo Effects

What we have just been discussing are the *specific* effects of chiropractic manipulation. Doubtless manipulation also has *non-specific* or placebo effects. Most treatments do. Placebo effects are the benefits felt by the patient simply because of the nature of the healing encounter—the drama of surgery, the magic potency of pills, the reassurance of the laying on of hands, the definitive "pop" of the chiropractic adjustment and the presence of a confident health professional.

A recent series of articles in *Lancet* reviewed placebo effects and concluded that they were the basis of treatment in former times, remain one of the most important elements of health care and should be embraced rather than rejected.[37] This was particularly so for chronic pain conditions which combined physical and psychological components. These, of course, are commonly seen in chiropractic practice.

G. What Is an Appropriate Course of Treatment with Manipulation?

The unanimous conclusion of a 1991 RAND Corporation expert panel reporting on *The Appropriateness of Spinal Manipulation for Low-Back Pain,* comprised of three chiropractors, two medical orthopedists, an internist, a family practitioner, a neurologist and an osteopath, was:

"An adequate trial of spinal manipulation is a course of two weeks for each of two different types of spinal manipulation (four weeks total) after which, in the absence of documented improvement, spinal manipulation is no longer indicated."[38]

Typically a patient is given manipulation three times weekly in initial weeks, then less frequently. This amounts to approximately 12 treatments over four weeks. This approach to frequency and duration of care has been endorsed in subsequent formal evidence-based chiropractic practice guidelines in the U.S.[39] and Canada.[40]

Some patients will only require one or a few treatments. If there is documented improvement after 4 weeks, but not complete relief of symptoms or restored function, the course of

manipulations may continue. Typically it should end within 8 weeks for uncomplicated conditions, within 16 weeks for other conditions unless there has been major trauma and/or complications.

For more on the appropriate frequency and duration of chiropractic treatment see Chapter 6, Section E, page 89.

References

1 Sandoz R. Some physical mechanisms and effects of spinal manipulation. Ann Swiss Chiropractic Assoc 1976;6:91–141.
2 Cassidy JD, Kirkaldy-Willis WH, Thiel HW. Chapter 16. In. Kirkaldy-Willis WH, Burton CV, eds. Managing low-back pain. 3rd ed. New York: Churchill Livingstone, 1992.
3 Mierau D, et al. Manipulation and mobilization of the third metacarpophalangeal joint: a quantitative radiographic and range of motion study. Man Med 1988;3:135–40.
4 Cassidy JD, Lopes AA, et al. The immediate effect of manipulation versus mobilization on pain and range of motion in the cervical spine: a randomized controlled trial. J Manip Physiol Ther 1992;15:570–5.
5 Hadler NM, Curtis P, et al. A benefit of spinal manipulation as adjunctive therapy for acute low-back pain: a stratified controlled trial. Spine 1987;12:703–6.
6 Spitzer WO, Skovron ML, et al. Scientific monograph of the Quebec task force on whiplash-associated disorders: redefining whiplash and its management. Spine 1995;20:8S.
7 Nilsson N, Christensen HW, et al. The effect of spinal manipulation in the treatment of cervicogenic headache. J Manip Physiol Ther 1997;2:326–30.
8 Hasselberg PD. Chiropractic in New Zealand, Report of the Commission of Inquiry. Wellington, New Zealand: Government Printer, 1979:130–31, 198.
9 Kenna C, Murtagh J. Spinal manipulation for doctors – a correspondence course, Unit 5. Aust Fam Phys 1985;14:453.
10 Grayson MF. Manipulation in back disorders. Br Med J 1986;293:1481–2.
11 Bourdillon J. Spinal Manipulation. 3rd ed. London, England: Heinemann Medical Books, 1982:24–5, 191.
12 Cyriax J. Textbook of orthopaedic medicine. Vol 2, 11th ed. London, England: Balliere Tindall, 1984:48,4.
13 Maigne R. Orthopedic medicine. Charles C. Thomas, Spingfield, IL, xi. 1972.
14 Lewit K. Manipulation - reflex therapy and/or restitution of impaired locomotor function. Man Med 1986;2:99–100.
15 Kirkaldy-Willis WH, Burton CV, eds. Managing low-back pain. 3rd ed. New York: Churchill Livingston, 1992.
16 Stoddard A. The Back – relief from pain. Canada: Prentice-Hall, 1979:17.
17 Melzack R, Wall PD. Pain mechanisms: a new theory. Science 1965:50–971.

18 Wyke B. Articular neurology and manipulative therapy. In Glasgow EF, Twomey LT, Scull ER, Kleynhans AM eds. Aspects of manipulative therapy. New York: Churchill Livingstone, 1985.

19 Herzog W, Scheele D, Conway PH. Electromyographic responses of back and limb muscles associated with spinal manipulative therapy. Spine 1999;24(2):146–53.

20 Giles LGF. Lumbo-sacral and cervical zygapophyseal joint inclusions. Man Med 1986;2:89–92.

21 Korr IM. Sustained sympathicotonia as a factor in disease. In: Korr IM, ed. The neurologic mechanisms in manipulative therapy. New York: Plenum Press, 1978.

22 Giles LGF. A histological investigation of human lower lumbar intervertebral canal (foramen) dimensions. J Manip Physiol Ther 1994;17:4–14.

23 Kirkaldy-Willis WH, Cassidy JD. Spinal manipulation in the treatment of low-back pain. Can Fam Phys 1985;31:535–40.

24 Cohen E, Triano J, et al. Biomechanical performance of spinal manipulation therapy by newly trained vs practicing providers: does experience transfer to unfamiliar procedures? J Manip Physiol Ther 1995;18:347–52.

25 Cassidy JD, Quon JA, et al. The effect of manipulation on pain and range of motion in the cervical spine: a pilot study. J Manip Physiol Ther 1992;15:495–500.

26 Terrett ACJ, Vernon H. Manipulation and pain tolerance. Am J Phys Med 1984;63:217–25.

27 Vernon T, Aker P, et al. Pressure pain threshold evaluation of the effect of spinal manipulation in the treatment of chronic neck pain: a pilot study. J Manip Physiol Ther 1990;13:13–6.

28 Shambaugh P. Changes in electrical activity in muscles resulting from chiropractic adjustment: a pilot study. J Manip Physiol Ther 1987;10:300–4.

29 Dishman D, Ploutz-Synder R, Bubulian R. Transient suppression of motoneural excitability following active or sham lumbosacral spinal manipulation measured by H-reflex amplitude. Proceedings of the International Conference on Spinal Manipulation. Vancouver, British Columbia, Canada: Foundation for Chiropractic Education and Research, 1998;193–5.

30 Harris W, Wagnon RJ. The effects of chiropractic adjustments on distal skin temperature. J Manip Physiol Ther 1987;10:57–60.

31 Fujimoto T, Budgell, B et al. Arterial tonometry in the measurement of the effects of innocuous mechanical stimulation of the neck on heart rate and blood pressure, J Auto Nerv Sys. 1999;75:109–115.

32 Yates RG, Lamping DL, et al. Effects of chiropractic treatment on blood pressure and anxiety: a randomized, controlled trial. J Manip Physiol Ther 1988;11:484–8.

33 Dhami MSI, Coyle BA, et al. Evidence for sympathetic neuron stimulation by cervicospinal manipulation. In: Proceedings of the first annual Conference on Research and Education. Sacramento, California: Pacific Consortium for Chiropractic Research, California Chiropractic Association 1986; A5 1–5.

34 Vernon HT, Dhami MSI, et al. Spinal manipulation and beta-endorphin: a controlled study of the effect of a spinal manipulation on plasma beta-endorphin levels in normal males. J Manip Physiol Ther 1986;9:115–23.

35 Brennan PC, Triano JJ, et al. Enhanced neutrophil respiratory burst as a biological marker for manipulation forces: duration of the effect and association with substance P and tumor necrosis factor. J Manip Physiol Ther 1992;15:83–9.

36 Briggs L, Boone WR. Effects of a chiropractic adjustment on changes in pupillary diameter: a model for evaluating somatovisceral response. J Manip Physio Ther 1988;11:181–9.

37 Weekly from October 1994 commencing with Thomas KB. The placebo in general practice. Lancet 1994;344:1066–7.

38 Shekelle PG, Adams AH, et al. The appropriateness of spinal manipulation for low-back pain: indications and ratings by a multidisciplinary expert panel. Santa Monica, California: RAND, 1991:Monograph No. R-4025/2—CCR/FCER

39 Haldeman S, Chapman-Smith D, Petersen DM, eds. Guidelines for chiropractic quality assurance and practice parameters. Proceedings of the Mercy Center Consensus Conference. Gaitersburg, Maryland: Aspen Publishers; 1993:179–84.

40 Henderson DJ, et al, eds. Clinical guidelines for chiropractic practice in Canada. JCCA 1994;38(1S).

41 Kirkaldy-Willis WH, Bernard TN, eds. Managing low-back pain. 4th ed. New York: Churchill Livingston, 1999.

CHAPTER 8

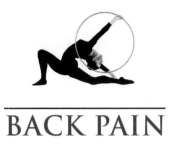

BACK PAIN

A. Introduction

It is probably no exaggeration to say that the chiropractic profession exists today, and has grown to such strength and numbers, because of its very successful management of patients with back pain.

Surveys consistently show that the majority of chiropractic patients have back pain—about 2 out of 3 (68%) according to a of UCLA/RAND study recently published in the *American Journal of Public Health*.[1] In the U.S. and Canada approximately 1 in 3 people who consult a health professional for back pain choose a chiropractor.[2]

There is now good evidence of the effectiveness and cost-effectiveness of chiropractic treatment, and independent patient surveys report a high level of patient satisfaction, far higher than for treatment of back pain by medical doctors.

In 1993 the Government of Ontario in Canada commissioned health economists at the University of Ottawa to review and report on the large body of international evidence on chiropractic management of back pain. Their conclusion:

"In our view, the constellation of the evidence of:

a. the effectiveness and cost-effectiveness of chiropractic management of low-back pain.

b. the untested, questionable or harmful nature of many current medical therapies.

c. the economic efficiency of chiropractic care for low-back pain compared with medical care.

d. the safety of chiropractic care.

e. the higher satisfaction levels expressed by patients of chiropractors

together offers an overwhelming case in favor of much greater use of chiropractic services in the management of low-back pain."[3]

This conclusion in the *Manga Report* was subsequently accepted by the government[4]. On safety and effectiveness, it was endorsed the following year by government-sponsored practice guidelines in the U.S.[5] and the U.K.[6] that are discussed in this chapter. (See Section C, pages 109–113.)

Because the management of back pain is such a major aspect of chiropractic practice, because the medical profession's approach to treatment of back pain patients is currently undergoing fundamental change, and because back pain has such huge cost to individuals and society as a whole, a full chapter of this book is now devoted to back pain.

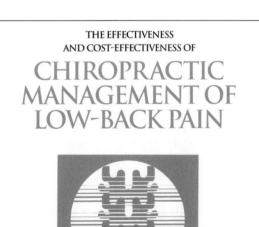

THE EFFECTIVENESS
AND COST-EFFECTIVENESS OF

CHIROPRACTIC
MANAGEMENT OF
LOW-BACK PAIN

PRAN MANGA, PH.D.
DOUG ANGUS, M.A.
COSTA PAPADOPOULOS, MHA
WILLIAM SWAN, B.A.

FUNDED BY THE ONTARIO MINISTRY OF HEALTH

The 1993 Manga Report from Canada

B.   Facts About Back Pain

During the past 20 years numerous articles on back pain published in medical journals have drawn attention to these facts:

1. *Back pain is very common.* Eighty-five percent of people will be disabled by an attack of back pain during their lives, and at any given time 7% of the adult population is suffering from a bout of back pain lasting 2 weeks or longer.[7]

   Back pain is the second most common reason, after respiratory disorders, that patients

Back pain is the most frequent and expensive health care problem in the 30–50 age group, and it the most common cause of work loss and disability.

   use the health care system.[8] It is now known that back pain is common from early adolescence—a new Danish study reports a large increase during the ages 12–14, and that 50% of young women have had their first episode of back pain by age 18, 50% of young men by age 20.[9]

2. *Most back pain is caused by mechanical problems in joints and muscles.* Over 90% of back pain, including strains and sprains and back pain caused by the normal wear and tear of life, is caused by *functional pathology* (e.g. restricted joint movements; stiffness, weakness or trigger points in muscle; nerve entrapment) rather than *structural pathology* (e.g. disease, tumors, fractures, disc herniation).[10]

3. *Back pain is very disabling and costly.* Back pain is the most frequent and expensive health care problem in the 30–50 age group, and it the most common cause of work loss and disability.[11] In North America workers' compensation boards report that 30% of claims are for back strain/sprain injuries, more than twice as many as any other category, and that these account for 50–60% of total cost because of the extremely high cost of chronic back injuries.[12] In 1985 U.S. workers' compensation boards disbursed $6 billion for low-back pain.[13]

4. *Disability and cost caused by back pain have been growing far more quickly than the population for decades and now represent an epidemic.* Between 1971 and 1981 the U.S. population rose by 12.5% but the population

disabled by back pain grew by 168%—14 times faster than the population.[14]

In the U.K. episodes of disability per 1,000 people per year rose dramatically from 1954/55 (21.7 for men, 8 for women) to 1980/81 (58.2 for men, 44.7 for women) and in the same period, days of sick certification rose for men by approximately 350% (506 to 1,882 days) and for women by approximately 500% (329 to 1,062).[15] By 1993 many experts and the World Health Organization recognized this sharply increasing disability from back pain as an epidemic.[16]

5. *Back pain has not been well understood and managed under traditional medical care.* For example:

   a) "Low-back pain treatment has represented the least cost-effective expenditure of health care dollars that the author is aware of." Charles Burton, MD, neurosurgeon, Minneapolis.[17]

   b) "We have not been honest with ourselves in the past when we have supported months of passive modality care that can offer no long-term benefit. We have not been fair to our patients when we have focused on *pain* rather than *function*. We, as medical clinicians, have relied only on the science available to us for the care of *structural deficits* . . . the time has come to develop rational principles of care." Vert Mooney, MD, orthopedic surgeon, San Diego.[18]

   c) "Modern medicine can successfully treat many serious spinal diseases and persisting nerve compression but has completely failed to cure the vast majority of patients with simple low-back pain . . .

   There is no evidence that rest has any beneficial effect on the natural history of low-back pain. On the contrary, there is strongly suggestive evidence that rest, particularly prolonged bed rest, may be the most harmful treatment ever devised and a potent cause of iatrogenic disability (*i.e. the treatment causes the disability).*" Gordon Waddell, MD, orthopedic surgeon, Glasgow.[19]

   d) "The conventional wisdom is that herniated discs are responsible for low-back pain, and that sacroiliac joints do not move significantly and do not cause low-back pain or dysfunction.

The ironic reality may well be that sacro-iliac joint dysfunctions are the major cause of low-back dysfunction, as well as the primary factor causing disc space degeneration and ultimate herniation of disc material."[20] Joseph Shaw, MD, orthopedic surgeon, Topeka.

C. The New Medical Approach to Back Pain

Since the early 1990s there has been a fundamental change in medical management of patients with low-back pain, broadly adopted since the publication of authoritative national practice guidelines in the U.S.[5] and the U.K.[6] in 1994.

These guidelines, government-sponsored and developed by multidisciplinary expert panels, change the approach to management for most patients, those with common or mechanical back pain, from rest and "wait-and-see" to maintaining daily activities and earliest possible rehabilitation. The first line of treatment is manipulation and simple non-prescription medication, and the guidelines encourage family physicians to refer patients for skilled manipulation.

As a result there is new common ground between the chiropractic and medical professions, each of which has a complementary and important role.

Gordon Waddell, quoted above and a prominent figure in the development of both the U.S. and U.K. guidelines, has been a significant force in changing the medical approach to managing low-back pain (LBP). In the mid-1980s he went to the Gulf state of Oman, helping to introduce new Western orthopedic services. He found LBP as common in Oman as anywhere else, but no-one was disabled—no-one stopped daily life or went to bed. Once Western care was fully introduced people in Oman adopted rest and stopped normal activities and there was now disability as well as back pain.

His subsequent paper in *Spine* in 1987, titled *A New Clinical Model for the Treatment of Low-Back Pain*,[19] won the Volvo Award as the best clinical science paper on the spine that year. His main arguments, since accepted, were:

- Most common LBP arises from functional pathology (mechanical problems of the joints and muscles) rather than structural pathology (fractures, disc herniation and other structural abnormalities seen on x-ray/imaging).

- Rest is not only inappropriate but is also harmful. Adverse effects include slower healing, demineralization of bone and 3% loss of muscle strength per day, decreased physical fitness, increased psychologic distress and depression, progressive loss of work habit and increased difficulty in starting rehabilitation.

- Helpful effects of early activity include promotion of bone and muscle strength, improved disc and cartilage nutrition, increased endorphin levels bringing reduced sensitivity to pain and avoidance of psychological problems.

- Medical management must change from rest to early activity. The model must change from one based on structural pathology and disease, to a *biopsychosocial model*. The various causes of most LBP include functional or mechanical pathology (*bio*), psychological factors (*psycho*) and factors related to lifestyle, work and how patients have learnt to view back pain (*social*).

From Waddell's paper in 1987 to 1994, during which time much new research on treatments for back pain was being published, there was a growing recognition of the need for

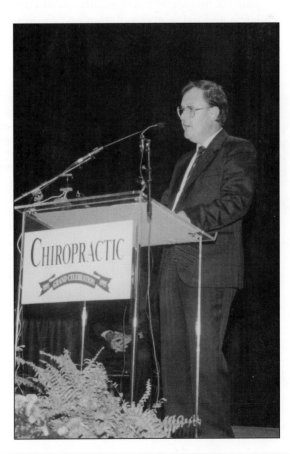

Orthopedic surgeon Dr. Gordon Waddell, shown here speaking at the Chiropractic Centennial Foundation Conference at the Convention Center, Washington, DC, July 1995.

change. This came with the new U.S.[5] and U.K.[6] guidelines in 1994. Most reviews of LBP since then have promoted these guidelines, which have now been adopted or followed by similar guidelines in a number of other countries.

Additionally there have now been updated guidelines in the U.K. by the Royal College of General Practitioners (RCGP), from an expert panel that included members of the medical, chiropractic, osteopathic and physiotherapy professions.[21] These RCGP guidelines are based on the international literature to October 1996.

Main components of all these guidelines, which are consistent, are:

1. The initial diagnosis should screen for "red flags"—specific pathology such as fracture, metastatic cancer and other disease processes that require medical care. A good patient history and physical examination will generally identify these patients, and resource intensive imaging and other studies are not encouraged unless the patient fails to progress in the first 4 weeks.

2. With the more than 90% of patients who do not have such red flags, the first line of management should be keeping the patient mobile and performing usual daily activities as much as possible, giving reassurance that pain felt on movement may hurt but will not harm and using manipulation and/or non-prescription medication for pain relief and return to normal function.

3. Specific exercise programs are not of proven value within the first 6 weeks for patients with acute pain. However they should be introduced once the acute pain has gone, especially for patients with a history of back pain. Exercises will prevent future episodes of pain, but only if continued on a regular basis for over 6 months—they should become a lifetime habit.

4. Bedrest should only be used for patients with extreme back and/or leg pain, and only then for a maximum of 2 to 3 days. It should be viewed as a temporary emergency measure, not as a treatment.

5. Non-prescription medications are preferred to prescription drugs because they are equally or more effective and have fewer side effects. Some prescription drugs have no evidence of effectiveness for back pain (e.g. anti-depressants and colchicine).

6. Physical modalities in common use for pain relief—ice, heat, short wave diathermy, ultrasound, TENS, traction, massage—have no evidence of producing a clinical effect and are not recommended as independent or principal treatments. (They may have a role

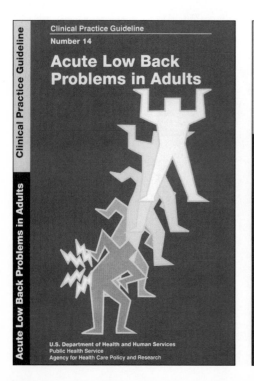

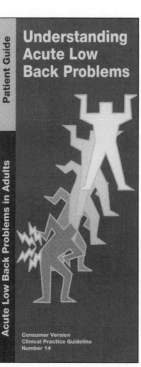

left: **Clinical Practice Guidelines from the U.S. (Agency for Health Care Policy and Research, DHHS, 1994) and** *right:* **the U.K. (Royal College of General Practitioners, 1996).**

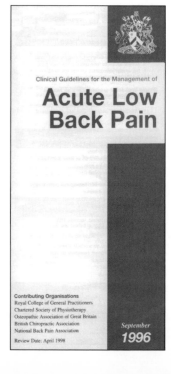

in combination with early activity, manipulation and exercises.)

7. There are recommendations against use of epidural, facet, ligamentous and trigger point injections.

8. Surgery should be used more narrowly and only after an appropriate trial of conservative treatments.

The main recommendations from the 1996 U.K. guidelines appear in Figure 1. The summary of the 1994 U.S. guideline published for health professionals appears in Figure 2.

TimeLife Medical has published a video titled *Low-Back Pain,* based on the 1994 U.S. guideline. It features medical and chiropractic experts and is one of a series of health videos available to the U.S. public through drugstores.

Figure 1 **Summary of U.K. 1994 Guidelines**

Principal Recommendations
U.K. Royal College of General Practitioners Clinical Guidelines for the Management of Acute Low-Back Pain September, 1996

Assessment
- Carry out diagnostic triage (*this means a differential diagnosis between simple backache, nerve root pain and possible serious spinal pathology*)
- X-rays are not routinely indicated in simple backache
- Consider psychosocial factors.

Drug Therapy
- Prescribe analgesics at regular intervals, not p.r.n.
- Start with paracetamol. If inadequate, substitute NSAIDs (e.g. ibuprofen or diclofenac) and then paracetamol-weak opioid compound (e.g. codydramol or coproxamol). Finally, consider adding a short course of muscle relaxant (e.g. diazepam or baclofen).

Bed Rest
- Do not recommend or use bed rest as a treatment of simple back pain.
- Some patients may be confined to bed for a few days as a consequence of their pain but this should not be considered a treatment.

Advice on Staying Active
- Advise patients to stay as active as possible and to continue normal daily activities
- Advise patients to increase their physical activities progressively over a few days or weeks.
- If a patient is working, then advice to stay at work or return to work as soon as possible is probably beneficial.

Manipulation
- Consider manipulative treatment within the first 6 weeks for patients who need additional help with pain relief or who are failing to return to normal activities.

Back Exercises
- Patients who have not returned to ordinary activities and work by 6 weeks should be referred for reactivation/rehabilitation

---

This 1996 TimeLife Medical video and personal workbook on back pain for the public incorporates the information from the U.S. AHCPR guidelines. The video is introduced by then U.S. Surgeon-General C. Everett Koop, and features chiropractic and medical doctors and their patients giving state-of-the-art advice on prevention and management of back pain.

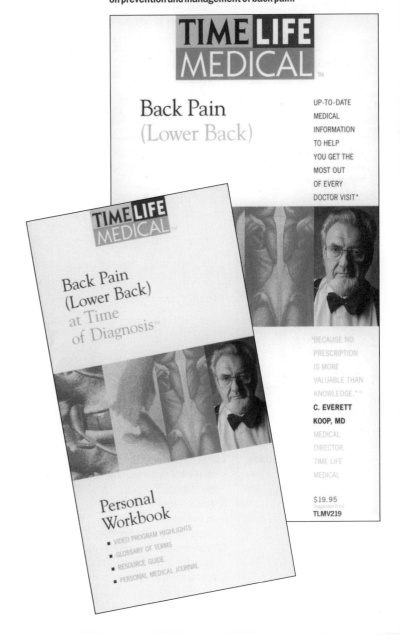

Figure 2 **Summary of U.S. 1994 Guidelines**

The ratings in parentheses indicate the scientific evidence supporting each recommendation according to the following scale:
A = strong research-based evidence (multiple relevant and high-quality scientific studies)
B = moderate research-based evidence (one relevant, high-quality scientific study or multiple adequate scientific studies)
C = limited research-based evidence (at least one adequate scientific study in patients with low back pain)
D = panel interpretation of evidence not meeting inclusion criteria for research-based evidence.
The number of studies meeting panel review criteria is noted for each category.

	Recommended	Option	Recommended Against
History and physical exam 34 studies	Basic history (B) History of cancer/infection (B) Signs/symptoms of cauda equina syndrome (C) History of significant trauma (C) Psychological history (C) Straight leg raising test (B) Focused neurological exam (B)	Pain drawing and visual analog scale (D)	
Patient education 14 studies	Patient education about low back symptoms (B) Back school in occupational settings (C)	Back school in non-occupational settings (C)	
Medication 23 studies	Acetaminophen (C) NSAIDs (B)	Muscle relaxants (C) Opioids, short course (C)	Opioids used >2 wks (C) Phenylbutazone (C) Oral steroids (C) Colchicine (B) Antidepressants (C)
Physical treatment methods 42 studies	Manipulation of low back during first month of symptoms (B)	Manipulation for patients with radiculopathy (C) Manipulation for patients with symptoms >1 month (C) Self-application of heat or cold to low back. Shoe insoles (C) Corset for prevention in occupational setting (C)	Manipulation for patients with undiagnosed neurologic deficits (D) Prolonged course of manipulation (D) Traction (B) TENS (C) Biofeedback (C) Shoe lifts (D) Corset for treatment (D)
Injections 26 studies		Epidural steroid injections for radicular pain to avoid surgery (C)	Epidural injections for back pain without radiculopathy (D) Trigger point injections (C) Ligamentous injections (C) Facet joint injections (C) Needle acupuncture (D)
Bed rest 4 studies		Bed rest of 2-4 days for severe radiculopathy (D)	Bed rest >4 days (B)
Activities and exercise 20 studies	Temporary avoidance of activities that increase mechanical stress on spine (D) Gradual return to normal activities (B) Low-stress aerobic exercise (C) Conditioning exercises for trunk muscles after 2 weeks (C) Exercise quotas (C)		Back-specific exercise machines (D) Therapeutic stretching of back muscles (D)

continued opposite

continued	Recommended	Option	Recommended Against
Detection of physiologic abnormalities 14 studies	If no improvement after 1 month, consider: Bone scan (C) Needle EMG and H-reflex tests to clarify nerve root dysfunction (C) SEP to assess spinal stenosis (C)		EMG for clinically obvious radiculopathy (D) Surface EMG and F-wave tests (C) Thermography (C)
X-rays of L-S spine 18 studies	When red flags for fracture present (C) When red flags for cancer or infection present (C)		Routine use in first month of symptons in absence of red flags (B) Routine oblique views (B)
Imaging 18 studies	CT or MRI when cauda equina, tumor, infection, or fracture strongly suspected (C) MRI test of choice for patients with prior back surgery (D) Assure quality criteria for imaging tests (B)	Myelography or CT-myelography for preoperative planning (D)	Use of imaging test before one month in absence red flags (B) Discography or CT-discography (C)
Surgical considerations 14 studies	Discuss surgical options with patients with persistent and severe sciatica and clinical evidence of nerve root compromise after 1 month of conservative therapy (B) Standard discectomy and microdiscectomy of similar efficacy in treatment of herniated disc (B) Chymopapain, used after ruling out allergic sensitivity, acceptable but less efficacious than discectomy to treat herniated disc (C)		Disc surgery in patients with back pain alone, no red flags, and no nerve root compression (D) Percutaneous discectomy less efficacious than chymopapain (C) Surgery for spinal stenosis within the first 3 months of symptoms (D) Stenosis surgery when justified by imaging test rather than patient's functional status (D) Spinal fusion during the first 3 months of symptoms in the absence of fracture, dislocation, complications of tumor or infection (C)
Psychosocial factors	Social, economic and psychological factors can alter patient response to symptoms and treatment (D)		Referral for extensive evaluation/treatment prior to exploring patient expectations or psychosocial factors (D)

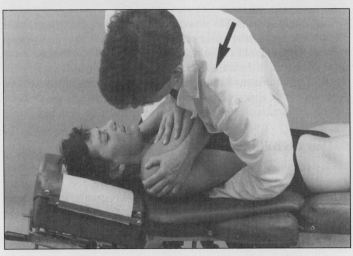

Manipulation of the mid-back. In this technique a quick adjustive force is applied downwards in the direction of the arrow. The chiropractor's left hand is placed under the sixth thoracic vertebra (T6)—in the position indicated by the block in the diagram. This gaps the joint at T5-T6.

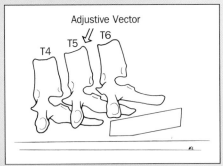

Adjustive Vector

T4   T5   T6

Mobilization of the low back. With this technique there is no sudden movement or force. Rotation is used to gap the joint between the third and fourth lumbar vertebrae.

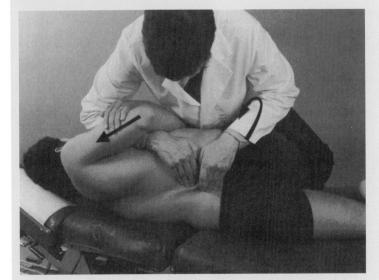

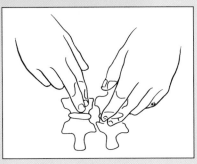

D. Chiropractic Management

1. **Diagnostic and Treatment Methods.** Chiropractors adopt the rehabilitation model now seen in medical practice guidelines. Management includes:

   a) *History and Examination.* A full history is followed by a physical exam that includes standard medical procedures (e.g. orthopedic and neurological tests, and the taking or ordering of x-rays and other imaging and laboratory tests where necessary) and specialized chiropractic tests (e.g. palpation of individual joints, muscles and other soft-tissues by hand to test for restricted ranges of motion and to provoke pain).

   Diagnosis. By education and law the scope of chiropractic practice, unlike physical therapy, includes diagnosis. Firstly a chiropractor has the responsibility of making a general diagnosis to find the presence of any disease or disorder that requires referral of the patient for medical care. Secondly there is a specific chiropractic diagnosis of joint and soft-tissue problems in the neuromusculoskeletal system. Psychosocial factors are also identified.

   b) *Treatment.* Goals of treatment are reduction of pain in the first few days, then restoring function to the neuromusculoskeletal system, preventing further loss of muscle tone (deconditioning) and preventing disability. This includes:

   • restoring normal joint mobility

   • inhibiting over-reactive musculature

   • improving muscular flexibility, coordination, strength and endurance

   • stretching retracted soft-tissues

   • propriosensory re-education (neuromuscular training on body position, balance, movement)

   • cardiovascular training

   • postural re-education

   Manual care includes joint manipulation (chiropractic adjustment), joint mobilization trigger point therapy and other soft-tissue techniques. Other treatment methods include physical therapy modalities (e.g. ice, heat, electrotherapy), rehabilitative exercises, orthotics and other supports and patient education on lifestyle (posture, nutrition, non-prescription medication, general exercise, work habits, managing other activities of daily living, etc.).

There is no use of prescription drugs, injections or surgery. However today it is quite usual for chiropractors to work in interdisciplinary practices where they provide post-operative care or, for example, manipulation under joint anesthesia administered by a medical colleague.[22]

How many treatments should a patient receive, and over how many weeks or months? These are matters of major importance and interest—they are dealt with at length in Chapter 6, "Scope of Practice" (see Section C, page 89 on Duration and Frequency of Care).

2. **Effectiveness**. Many studies have now confirmed the effectiveness of chiropractic manipulation, and chiropractic management generally, for patients with mechanical low-back pain (also called common, simple or non-specific back pain), the type of back-pain suffered by over 90% of patients.[23,24,25,26,27,28]

The most influential trial because of its size, scientific design, independence, and results has been one by Meade that was published in the *British Medical Journal* in 1990,[24] with long-term results published in 1995.[25] This trial was also important because it gave positive answers to two questions asked by many medical doctors:

- Are the benefits of chiropractic treatment long-term as well as short-term?

- Is chiropractic treatment valuable for patients with chronic pain—pain experienced for many months or years?

The trial was also important and unusual—though this feature is now being incorporated into many more trials—in that it directly compared two treatment methods *as they are given in normal day-to-day practice*. Usually trials have taken one aspect of treatment—a medication or a form of electro-therapy, manipulation, exercise, etc.—and given it in a standard and defined way to each patient. This has then been compared with another standardized treatment or a placebo/sham intervention such as a pill without medication or detuned diathermy.

This has some scientific advantages, but has the overall disadvantage that it gives information on the effectiveness of a treatment in circumstances that are very different from the way it is used in practice. This is a particular problem for physical treatments such as manipulation, which varies according to the need of each patient and is only one part of overall management, which includes other treatments, exercises and back education. The Meade trial compared chiropractic and medical management as actually experienced by patients in normal life. In summary:

- *Purpose.* The aim of the Meade study which was a large (741 patients), multi-center (11 pairs of clinics throughout the U.K.), randomized, controlled trial by medical researchers funded by the British Medical Research Council, was to compare standard chiropractic and medical/physiotherapy (hospital out-patient back pain clinics) treatment for patients with low-back pain of mechanical origin. Treatment was at the discretion of the treating practitioners—they could use their normal treatment approach, whatever that was—except that there was a maximum of 10 treatments and care was to be "concentrated in the first 3 months."

- *Treatment.* Virtually all patients receiving chiropractic care received joint manipulation and back education. Many also received exercises and/or physical therapy modalities. The great majority of hospital out-patients (84%) received manipulation or mobilization from physiotherapists according to the techniques of Cyriax or Maitland. Many also received one or more of traction, exercises, physical therapy modalities and corsets.

- *Results.* Measurement of results was objective (i.e. by a professional who did not know what treatment the patient had received—improvement in degrees of straight leg raise and lumbar spine flexion) and subjective (completion by the patient of a questionnaire on pain and ability to perform various functions—

the Oswestry Index) and was done at 6 weeks, 6 months, 1 year and 2 years (i.e. during and long after completion of treatment). The chiropractic patients did significantly better, including those with severe or chronic pain, and these superior results were maintained after 1 and 2 years.

Meade concluded that chiropractic treatment had long-term success in the management of patients with mechanical back pain, was highly cost-efficient

Medical and chiropractic authorities now agree that the treatment of back and/or leg pain from disc herniation by skilled manipulation is proven both safe and effective.

and should be funded within the British National Health System.

3. **Chronic Pain**. Patients with chronic or long-term pain have different needs than those with an acute attack of pain—as the result of the pain, its impact on their lives, and unsuccessful treatments, 50% of those with chronic pain have at least mild depression[29] and all have muscular weakness and imbalance. Psychosocial factors, particularly the ability to perform modified work and attitudes to work, are very important.

Evidence of the effectiveness of chiropractic care now includes studies by Meade[24,25] in the U.K., Triano in the U.S.,[30] and Kirkaldy-Willis and Cassidy in Canada.[27] For a recent text describing chiropractic management of chronic pain patients, see Liebenson's *Rehabilitation of the Spine: A Practitioner's Manual*.[31] Treatments include manipulation, rehabilitative exercises and education on posture, work habits and lifestyle.

No one disputes the effectiveness of chiropractic treatment for short-term or acute back pain but some medical doctors still question its value for long-term or chronic back pain. They would not if they were aware of current research. An eminent team of Dutch researchers, van Tulder, Koes and Bouter did a systematic review of all the trials of the most common treatments for acute and chronic back pain in 1996. This was published in the leading medical journal *Spine* in 1997 and they conclude:

"Strong evidence was found for the effectiveness of manipulation, back schools and exercise therapy for chronic low-back pain, especially for short-term effects."[32]

4. **Disc Herniation**. Medical and chiropractic authorities now agree that the treatment of back and/or leg pain from disc herniation by skilled manipulation is proven both safe and effective,[33,34] and that disc herniation should now be seen primarily as a non-surgical disease to be treated by conservative methods.[35] Key points include:

- Often a herniated disc is present, as confirmed by imaging, but the source of the pain is some other joint or muscle dysfunction. It is now known that approximately 40% of persons over the age of 40 have disc herniations clearly visible on imaging but no pain or other symptoms at all.[36]

- Where the disc is the source of the pain, the primary cause of the pain is not nerve root compression, as previously thought, but inflammation (from disc material that has escaped into the epidural space). Manipulation seems to reduce the inflammation, in some cases by moving the herniated material away from the nerve root. Nerve compression, when present, causes loss of sensation, motor power and reflexes rather than pain.

- Fear of harm from manipulation comes from a misunderstanding of the biomechanics of the lumbar spine (lowback). Researchers have shown that normal discs withstand an average of 23 degrees of rotation before damage from rotational stress, degenerated discs an average of 14 degrees. The joints of the lumbar spine (posterior facet joints) only allow 3 degrees of rotation on manipulation.[37] Cassidy, Thiel and Kirkaldy-Willis have concluded that in most circumstances "it is hard to comprehend how the small amount of rotation introduced during side posture manipulation could damage or irritate a healthy or herniated disc."

In the U.S. many medical doctors now routinely refer selected patients with lumbar disc herniations for chiropractic assessment and management, with the goals of alleviating pain and avoiding surgery. The following two case reports show excellent results—and also demonstrate that chiropractic management involves more than just manipulation:

- A 31 year old man California man with severe low-back and leg pain and a large L5-S1 disc herniation shown on MRI was referred by his physician for chiropractic management. This included the McKenzie protocol, manipulation, mobilization, trigger point therapy and rehabilitative exercises. The patient returned to modified work after 3 weeks, was discharged as asymptomatic after 20 visits over seven weeks, and on reassessment 6 months later had no significant symptoms or lifestyle restrictions.[38]

- A 36 year old New Mexico woman with a central/left disc herniation at L5-S1 shown on CT scan was referred by her physician for chiropractic management. She received 9 treatment sessions over a 3 week period each consisting of 4 treatments—interferential electrotherapy, lumbar spine manipulation, sacroiliac joint manipulation and flexion traction. She was also prescribed an orthotic and given instruction in stretching and strengthening exercises. There was consistent improvement throughout. After 9 sessions the patient returned to normal activities of daily living, including her jogging and exercise routine, with no ill effects. At 7 months follow-up she was symptom-free.[39]

5. **Sacroiliac Joint Dysfunction**. Back pain often results from dysfunction of the sacroiliac (SI) joints, which are found on each side of the pelvis at the base of the spine as shown in Figure 3. Many medical doctors were taught that the SI joints do not move so this has been a point of controversy. It is no longer controversial, and the foremost medical manipulators in North America describe the importance of the SI joints this way:

"The sacroiliac joint appears to be the single greatest cause of back pain. The range of motion is small and difficult to describe but, when normal joint play is lost, agonizing pain can be precipitated . . . (the sacroiliac joints) are complex and not fully understood, but it is clear to the authors that they can have a profound effect on body mechanics . . . anyone who still holds the view that these joints are immobile can never hope to achieve control of common back pain."[40]

6. **Safety.** Spinal manipulation for back pain is safe, as is confirmed by the U.S. and U.K. guidelines already discussed. One of the reasons it is recommended as a first line of treatment in these guidelines is that, in comparison with all medication, including non-prescription anti-inflammatories and analgesics, it has very few risks and side effects. There are of course a number of contraindications to manipulation, includ-

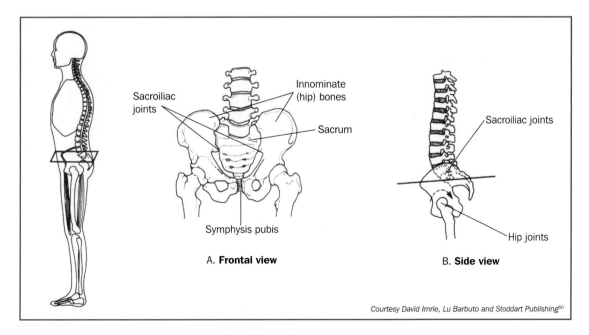

A. **Frontal view**   B. **Side view**

Courtesy David Imrie, Lu Barbuto and Stoddart Publishing[60]

Figure 3 **The Pelvic Ring and Sacroiliac Joints**

Figure 4.1 **Average Cost per Patient Under Workers' Compensation, Victoria, Australia, 1990-1991**

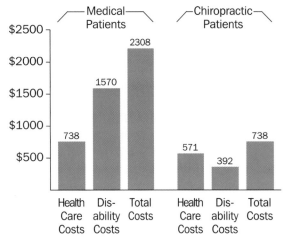

Figure 4.2 **Patients Developing Chronic Pain from Workplace Injuries, Victoria, Australia, 1990-1991**

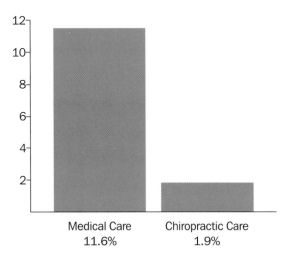

ing fracture, risk of fracture because of a condition such as advanced osteoporosis, and spinal instability, but these are all well-recognized. The subject of disc herniation has been dealt with above—herniation is not usually a contraindication for chiropractic care, but requires appropriate skill and modification of technique.

7. **Cost-effectiveness**. There is now a convincing body of evidence showing a 20–60% saving in total health care and compensation costs for employers, governments, and other third party payors when chiropractic care is substituted for medical care for patients with back pain.

The evidence is consistent and comes from worker's compensation studies in North America and Australia, clinical trials in various countries, individual employer experience and now sophisticated analysis of U.S. health insurance data by health economists. It is reviewed most thoroughly in two recent

reports from Manga and Angus,[3,41] health economists from the University of Ottawa in Canada (1993 and 1998). Only two studies suggest that chiropractic care is not more cost-effective than medical care, one by Carey[42] and the other by Shekelle.[43] These may be sound as medical research but, as Manga and Angus note, "have significant design problems from an economist's point of view."[41] Problems include poor matching of patients, failure to include all costs, invalid attribution of costs and inadequate sample size, and these problems render their conclusions unreliable. Rosner supports this criticism.[44]

The overall evidence shows:

a) There is a 20-60% savings in total costs (direct costs for health care, and indirect costs for disability and time off work) when a matched group of patients receives chiropractic care rather than medical care for back pain.

b) The actual primary treatment costs in the acute or initial stage are often higher for chiropractic care, because there is more intensive intervention. But this results in substantial savings in secondary health care costs (fewer specialist services, surgeries, hospitalizations) and compensation costs.

As to secondary health care costs, when a patient attends a medical doctor, the doctor's fees are only 23% of total health care cost —77% is cost of other diagnostic specialist and hospital services. With chiropractic care 80% of the cost is chiropractic fees—only 20% is secondary health care costs.[41]

c) However, the most significant area of cost savings under chiropractic care is in the cost of compensation for disability. Because of better earlier results, far fewer patients experience long-term (chronic) pain, time off work and disability under chiropractic care than under medical care.

The better designed workers' compensation studies show this quite dramatically. Jarvis[45] reported that workers in Utah with similar back injuries (identical ICD-9 codes) had approximately 10 times the number of days off work on average (20.7 versus 2.4) and compensation costs ($668.39 vs. $68.38) if they chose medical rather than chiropractic care.

Ebrall, looking at comparable injured workers in the State of Victoria, Australia[46] in the 1990-91 compensation year, reported average payments per claimant of $963.47 for chiropractic patients (health care cost $571.45, compensation cost $392.02) and $2,308.10 for medical patients (health care cost $738.17, compensation $1,569.93). The higher compensation costs for medical patients reflected the fact that more medical patients developed chronic pain (11.6%) than chiropractic patients (1.9%). These results are illustrated in Figure 4.

d) *A U.K. Workplace Study—Advantage to Individual Employers.* The *Journal of Occupational Health*[47] has recently reported a study in which two companies with 750 employees referred employees complaining of neck/arm or back/leg pain for chiropractic treatment over a period of two years in 1994/95. The companies subsidized the cost of care in expectation of better effectiveness, patient satisfaction and overall cost savings.

The results were rewarding—extremely high self-rated improvement and patient satisfaction, and an 18% net saving of costs in the first year (30% saving in disability/sickness payments, less 12% for the treatment costs subsidized) and approximately 40% net saving in the second year.

e) *Savings under Managed Care.* Even in a contemporary U.S. managed care environment, where there are protocols to control cost carefully, there may be substantial savings with chiropractic care for back and neck pain patients. Mosley[48] analyzed claims over 12 months in a Louisiana HMO in which patients were permitted direct access to either a primary gatekeeper MD or a participating doctor of chiropractic. Direct health care costs per chiropractic patient were only 70% of costs per medical patient over a range of identical ICD-9 diagnoses—in other words a saving of 30% or about one third. Clinical results were equivalent.

Surgical rates were similar in this instance, but medical patients received much more imaging and prescription drugs.

Health economists Johnson and Baldwin, in a recent well-designed study for Zenith Insurance of 850 California workers who completed an episode of back pain in the years 1991–1993, also concluded that "substantial savings" were possible from shifting the care of workers' compensation back patients to chiropractors.[49] Total claim costs were

Even in a contemporary U.S. managed care environment there may be substantial savings with chiropractic care for back and neck pain patients.

reduced by approximately 20% ($1,526 for chiropractic patients and $1,875 for medical patients) when workers with equivalent injuries chose chiropractic care. Most of the savings came from earlier return to work and lower indemnity costs.

f) *Medstat Data Analysis.* Most evidence, Manga and Angus point out, fails to capture all of the relevant costs. If it did so the advantage for chiropractic care would be even greater. Full costs per episode of care include all health care costs, compensation costs, and other indirect costs incurred by patients and/or their families and employers. A strict analysis of health care costs would include the cost of side effects and iatrogenic costs (costs arising from harm from the treatment, which can be very significant in the area of back pain—e.g. subsequent surgeries and/or long-term reliance on medications after an initial failed surgery.)

In their view, the best evidence on complete health care costs appears in two recent papers by Stano and Smith,[50,51] U.S. health economists, analyzing records from the Michigan health benefits consulting firm MedStat Systems Inc. which covers 2 million patients across the U.S. Their analysis is for the 2 year period July 1988 to June 1990. In summary:

i) The studies look at chiropractic and

medical use and costs for 208 ICD-9 code diagnoses for various conditions in patients who were equally free to choose medical or chiropractic care for these conditions under the terms of their employment health benefits plans. The entire claims history and all costs for these patients were known.

ii) After regression analysis to ensure matching populations in all material respects (e.g. severity of complaints, age, sex, location, relation to insur-

Common reasons for higher satisfaction with chiropractic care included more information received about the back problems, cause of pain, recovery from pain, content of care and instructions on exercise, posture and lifting.

ance plan—employee or dependent, insurance plan type—similar access to, and similar deductibles for chiropractic and medical care, etc.), the study group was 7,077 patients.

iii) Medical care costs were significantly higher. For the 9 high-frequency codes most typically used by both chiropractic and medical doctors, mostly involving back and sacroiliac disorders including disc degeneration and sciatica, medical payments were 47% higher for outpatient care, 61% higher for total care.

g) *Substitution and Complementary Care.* Chiropractic and medical care may be *substitutes* for each other for many patients with back pain, but also have a *complementary role.*

Some patients, most obviously those with internal injuries, disease, back fractures or requiring surgery, fall outside the scope of chiropractic practice and require referral if they consult a chiropractor. Similarly, medical doctors now refer many patients with mechanical back pain to chiropractors for manipulation and rehabilitation. Manga and Angus, as health economists, point out that protocols for timely referral of patients have a major impact on cost.

They also indicate that true substitution of services is a key factor in realizing

potential savings. This is achievable as many of the studies show. But it requires strength of purpose, often fighting vested interests. To quote Manga and Angus:

"Huge savings are certain if substitutions are carefully implemented . . . there are literally dozens of studies pointing to evidence-based manpower substitution, but for a variety of professional, political, insurance practice and other administrative reasons, many of these human health resources substitutions have yet to occur."[52]

8. **Patient Satisfaction**. A dramatic change in recent years is that this aspect of health care, representing the consumer's overall assessment of the quality of the health services received and the professionals who provide them, has moved from the wings to center stage. Reasons include increased patient education and rights, improved choice in health care and the growth of third party payment and management.

Patient satisfaction with chiropractic services generally is discussed in Chapter 9, "Public and Medical Attitudes Towards Chiropractic" (see page 128). With respect to back pain there is evidence from independent studies and polls that patients are generally very satisfied with chiropractic management, much more so than with medical management. The studies to 1993 are reviewed in the *Manga Report*[3] and they are supported by more recent studies.[41]

The most thorough comparative study dealt with 457 back pain patients at a Washington HMO who had visited either family physicians (215 patients) or chiropractors (242 patients). This study looked at specific causes of satisfaction or dissatisfaction and found:

a) The percentage of chiropractic patients who were "very satisfied" with the care they received for low-back pain was 3 times that of patients of family physicians—66% versus 22%.

b) Common reasons for higher satisfaction with chiropractic care included:

- More information received about the back problems, including the cause of pain, recovery from pain, content of care and instructions on exercise, posture and lifting.

- Amount of time listening to their description of the pain.

- Belief that the pain was real and an expression of concern.

- Confidence in the diagnosis and effectiveness of treatment.[53]

9. **Access to Chiropractic Care.** There is now strong independent evidence that chiropractic treatment for patients with back pain is effective, cost-effective, satisfying to patients and now consistent with the best medical practice. But is it available?

The answer to this question, in a world where patients increasingly expect their health care to be subsidized by their employers or the government and where medical care for back pain generally is, depends upon:

i) Organization of health care services—does the managed care or other health care plan from which you get your health care include chiropractic services.

ii) Funding arrangements—is the cost of chiropractic treatment covered to the same extent as medical treatment.

This has recently been demonstrated once more by a U.K. study.[54] When the 1994 government-sponsored U.K. back pain guidelines recommended skilled manipulation as a primary approach to treatment the Wiltshire Health Authority, a government-funded regional health authority in England, provided funding for "manipulation services" in a pilot project to see if there were benefits if general medical practitioners (GPs) followed the new guidelines. The results are of interest:

a) The study compared a group of 194 patients treated in 11 GP practices between July and October 1995, and a second group of 344 patients treated in the same practices from November 1995 to March 1996—the important difference was that funding was available for "manipulation services" in accordance with the U.K. guidelines in the second period.

b) There was a major shift in medical referral patterns. In the earlier group only 2% of the back pain patients were referred for manipulation (2% to chiropractors, 0% to osteopaths), while in the latter group 53% were referred (28% to chiropractors, 25% to osteopaths). Referrals for physiotherapy services, funded at all relevant times, went down from 72% to 21%.

c) Results of this "substantial shift of referrals to manipulation practitioners" included fewer referrals to secondary care; fewer GP consultations; less drug use; and fewer certified sickness days—"demonstrable savings in sickness incapacity benefits were evident."

10. **The Problem of Over-Treatment.** There are chiropractors who are guilty of over-treatment, some to a gross and fraudulent degree, and they are an embarrassment to the profession. If you are in the United States, Canada, Australia or other countries where the practice of chiropractic is regulated you should report any case of obvious over-treatment to the state/provincial regulatory body for disciplinary action.

Although it somehow seems to be more newsworthy when chiropractors are at fault, there is no evidence that over-treatment is a more common problem for them than other health professions. Actually, as a matter of logic, there would not be the strong evidence of cost-effectiveness and patient satisfaction already discussed in this chapter if over-treatment was widespread. When the television program *20/20* aired a segment on Medicaid over-treatment and fraud by chiropractors in Michigan and Nebraska in 1998, the Medicaid officer interviewed affirmed that this type of behavior was disgraceful but limited to a few individuals and not representative of the profession.

What is an appropriate course of chiropractic treatment, both as to duration and frequency of care? This is something on which the profession has established formal clinical guidelines. These have been discussed in Section E, Chapter 6—see page 90. A RAND Corporation study has also provided a guideline on what amounts to an adequate trial of spinal manipulation—see Section G, Chapter 7, page 105.

11. **The Natural Remission Myth.** The principle of natural remission is that most patients with low-back pain seen in general medical practice will get better without any treatment within a month anyway—the problem

will remit or resolve naturally. This, together with difficulty in establishing an exact cause or diagnosis for back pain, has been the basis of the medical approach of bed rest, medication for pain and "let's wait and see."

Recent research in the UK, studying the general population[55] and nurses,[56] shows that the concept of high rates of natural remission is wrong—it is a myth based on misinterpretation of earlier evidence. British medical epidemiologists Croft et al. decided to investigate the concept of natural remission because it was logically inconsistent with other data on back pain. In the UK for example:

- 38% of adults report a significant episode of low-back pain each year. (This suggests that many have a recurring unsolved problem.)

- The fact that a person has a previous episode of low-back pain is the strongest risk factor for a new episode.

- The prevalence of disabling low-back pain for which benefits are paid has risen greatly in recent decades.

They found that the concept of natural remission was based on a 1973 study of one medical practice where recovery was judged on whether or not patients made further visits to the general practitioner, not on whether the patient actually got better.

Croft et al. did a much more thorough study following all adults with low-back pain consulting two general medical practices in Manchester over 12 months. Of 463 patients with a new episode of low-back pain 275 (59%) did not have a further GP consultation after the first visit, and only 38 (8%) had a repeat visit after 3 months.

However all patients were visited by a research nurse within a week of their first consultation and again after 3 and 12 months. Standard measurements of pain and disability were taken. Although most patients did not return after the first visit, only 21% had recovered within three months, and only 25% by 12 months.

A final and important statistic was this: of those patients disabled by pain at the first visit, only 18%—less than 1 in 5—had fully recovered by 12 months.

In other words, there is not a high natural remission rate. Croft et al. conclude that their profession has been wrong on this. Patients with low-back pain should not be seen as having mainly short-term problems, most of which get better, and a small number of long-term chronic problems. Rather, low-back pain "should be viewed as a chronic problem with an untidy pattern of grumbling symptoms and periods of relative freedom from pain and disability, interspersed with acute episodes, exacerbations and recurrences."

Experts such as neurologist Dr. Scott Haldeman, Past-President of the North American Spine Society, and orthopedic surgeon Dr. Vert Mooney, Past-President, International Society for the Study of the Lumbar Spine, agree.[57,58] Common or mechanical low-back pain is not something that fully resolves or is cured by treatment, whether by medical doctors, chiropractors or anyone else. It is a recurring condition in people who have developed a weakness but are getting on with their lives.

The goal of management is to limit disability and pain as promptly and as effectively as possible, and to try to prevent future problems through education, exercise and preventive care.

References

1   Hurwitz EL, Coulter ID, et al. Use of chiropractic services from 1985 through 1991 in the United States and Canada. Am J Pub Health 1998;8:771–6

2   Carey TS, Evans AT, et al. Acute severe low-back pain: a population-based study of prevalence and care-seeking. Spine 1996;21:339–44.

3   Manga P, Angus D, et al. The effectiveness and cost-effectiveness of chiropractic management of low-back pain. Ottawa, Ontario: Pran Manga and Associates, University of Ottawa, 1993.

4   Chiropractic services review committee report. Ontario Ministry of Health, 1994:Chapter 1.

5   Bigos S, Bowyer O, Braen G, et al. Acute low-back problems in adults. Clinical practice guideline no. 14. Rockville, Maryland: Agency for Health Care Policy and Research, Public Health Service, U.S. Department of Health and Human Services, 1994; AHCPR Publication No. 95-0642.

6   Rosen M, Breen A, et al. Management guidelines for back pain. Appendix B In: Report of a clinical standards advisory group committee on back pain. London, England: Her Majesty's Stationery Office (HMSO), 1994.

7   Deyo R. Descriptive epidemiology of low-back pain and its related medical care in the United States. Spine 1987;12:264-8.

8 Deyo RA , Cherkin DC, Conrad D, Volinn E. Cost controversy crisis: low-back pain and the health of the public. Ann Rev of Pub Health 1991;12:141–56.

9 Leboeuf-Yde C, Kyvik KO. At what age does low-back pain become a common problem? A study of 29,424 individuals aged 12-41 years. Spine 1998;23:228–34.

10 Kirkaldy-Willis WH, Bernard TN, eds. Managing low-back pain. 4th edition. New York: Churchill Livingston, 1999.

11 Spengler, et al. Back injuries in industry: a retrospective study part I overview and cost analysis. Spine 1986;11:241–5.

12 Burton CV. In: Mooney V, ed. Symposium on evaluation and care of lumbar spine problems. Ortho Clin N Am 1983;14:539.

13 Frymoyer JW, Mooney V. Current concepts review: occupational orthopaedics. J Bone Joint Surg 1986;68A:469–73.

14 Prevalence of selected impairments, United States 1971. Hyattsville, Maryland: National Center for Health Statistics 1975; DHHS Publication No. (PHS)75-1526 (Series 10, No. 99); 1981 DHHS Publication No. (PHS)87-1587 (Series 10, No. 159).

15 Waddell G. A new clinical model for the treatment of low-back pain. Spine 1987;12:632–44.

16 Mikheev M. Opening Address, 1993 World Chiropractic Congress. London, England: Office of Occupational Health, World Health Organization, May 27, 1993.

17 Burton C. Conservative management of low-back pain. Postgrad Med 1981;70:168–85.

18 Mooney V. Foreword. In: Mayer TG, Gatchel RJ. Functional restoration for spinal disorders: the sports medicine approach. Philadelphia, Pennsylvania: Lea and Febiger, 1988.

19 Ref 15, Supra.

20 Shaw JL. The role of the sacroiliac joint as a cause of low-back pain and dysfunction in low-back pain and its relation to the sacroiliac joint. Vleeming A, Mooney V, Snijders C, Dorman T, eds. Proceedings of the First Interdisciplinary World Congress on Low-back Pain and its Relation to the Sacroiliac Joint. San Diego, California: University of California, November 5-6, 1992.

21 Waddell G, Feder G, et al. Low-back pain evidence review. London, England: Royal College of General Practitioners, 1996.

22 Lawrence DC. Chapter 2 in Advances in Chiropractic. Vol. 4., Michaelson MR, Dreyfuss PH. Manipulation under Joint Anesthesia/Analgesia: A Proposed Interdisciplinary Treatment Approach for Recalcitrant Spinal Axis Pain of Synovial Joint Origin. St Louis, Missouri: Mosby Yearbook 2, 1997.

23 Hadler NM, Curtis P, et al. A benefit of spinal manipulation as adjunctive therapy for acute low-back pain: a stratified controlled trial. Spine 1987;12:703–6.

24 Meade TW, Dyer S, et al. Low-back pain of mechanical origin: randomised comparison of chiropractic and hospital outpatient treatment. Br Med J 1990;300:1431–7.

25 Meade TW, Dyer S, et al. Randomised comparison of chiropractic and hospital outpatient management for low-back pain: results from extended follow up. Br Med J 1995;311:349–51.

26 Shekelle PG, Adams AH, et al. The appropriateness of spinal manipulation for low-back pain: project overview and literature review. Santa Monica, California: RAND, 1991; Monograph No. R-4025/1—CCR/FCER.

27 Kirkaldy-Willis WH, Cassidy JD. Spinal manipulation in the treatment of low-back pain. Can Fam Phys 1985;31:535–40.

28 Bronfort G. Efficacy of manual therapies of the spine. Amsterdam: Vrije Universiteit EMGO Institute, 1997.

29 Carroll L. Psychological problems encountered in chiropractic clinical practice. In: Lawrence DJ, ed. Advances in chiropractic. Vol. 4. Baltimore, Maryland: Mosby, 1997; 155-80.

30 Triano JJ, McGregor M, et al. Manipulative therapy versus education programs in chiropractic low-back pain. Spine 1995;20:948–55.

31 Liebenson C. Rehabilitation of the spine: a practitioner's manual. Baltimore, Maryland: Williams & Wilkins, 1996.

32 van Tulder MW, Koes BW, Bouter LX. Conservative treatment of acute and chronic nonspecific low-back pain. Spine 1997;22:2128–56.

33 Cassidy JD, Thiel HW, Kirkaldy-Willis KW. Side posture manipulation for lumbar intervertebral disc herniation. J Manip Physiol Ther 1993;16:96–103.

34 Nwuga VCB. Relative therapeutic efficacy of vertebral manipulation and conventional treatment in back pain management. Am J Phys Med 1982;6:273–278.

35 Bozzao A, Gallucci M, et al. Lumbar disc herniation: MR Imaging assessment of natural history in patients treated without surgery. Neuroradiol 1992;185:135–41.

36 Wiesel SW. A study of computer-assisted tomography: the incidence of positive CAT scans in an asymptomatic group of patients. Spine 1984;9:549–51.

37 Ref 33, Supra.

38 Morris CE. Chiropractic rehabilitation of a patient with SI radiculopathy associated with a large lumbar disc herniation. J Manip Physiol Ther 1999;22:38–44.

39 Crawford MC. Chiropractic management of acute low-back pain. Alt Ther 1999;5:112.

40 Bourdillon JF, Day EA. Spinal manipulation. 4th ed. London, England: William Heinemann Medical Books, 1987:229.

41 Manga P, Angus D. Enhanced chiropractic coverage under OHIP as a means of reducing health care costs, attaining better health outcomes and improving the public's access to cost-effective health services. Ontario, Canada: University of Ottawa, 1998.

42 Carey TS, Garrett J, et al. The outcomes of care for acute low-back pain among patients seen by primary care practitioners, chiropractors and orthopedic surgeons. New Engl J Med 1995;333:913–7.

43 Shekelle PG, Markovich M, et al. Comparing the costs between provider types of episodes of back pain care. Spine 1995;20: 221–7.

44 Rosner AL. Letter to the Editor. Spine 1995;20:2395–8.

45 Jarvis KB, Phillips RB, et al. Cost per case comparison of back injury of chiropractic versus medical management for conditions with identical diagnosis codes. J Occup Med 1991;33:847–52.

46 Ebrall PS. Mechanical low-back pain: a comparison of medical and chiropractic management within the Victorian workcare scheme. Chiro J Aust 1992;22:47–53.

47 Jay TC, Jones SL, et al. A chiropractic service arrangement for musculoskeletal complaints in industry: a pilot study. Occup Med 1998;48:389–95.

48 Mosley CD, Cohen IG, et al. Cost-effectiveness of chiropractic care in a managed care setting. Am J Managed Care 1996;11:280–2.

49 Johnson W, Baldwin M. Why is the treatment of work related injuries so costly? New evidence from California. Inquiry 1996;33:56–65.

50 Stano M, Smith M. Chiropractic and medical costs for low-back care. Med Care 1996;34:191–204.

51 Smith M, Stano M. Cost and recurrences of chiropractic and medical episodes of low-back care. J Manip Physiol Ther 1997;20:5–12.

52 Manga P, Angus D, et al. The effectiveness and cost-effectiveness of chiropractic management of low-back pain. Ontario, Canada: Pran Manga and Associates, University of Ottawa, 1993:65–70.

53 Cherkin DC, McCornack FA. Patient evaluations of low-back pain care from family physicians and chiropractors. West J Med 1989;50:351–5.

54 Scheurmier N, Breen AC. A pilot study of the purchase of manipulation services for acute low-back pain in the United Kingdom. J Manip Physiol Ther 1998;21:14–8.

55 Croft PR, Macfarlane GJ et al. Outcome of low back pain in general practice: a prospective study. Br Med J: 316:1356–1359.

56 Smedley J, Inskip H et al. Natural history of low back pain: a longitudinal study in nurses. Spine 1998;23(22):2422–2426.

57 Haldeman S. Personal communication, August 2, 1998.

58 Mooney V. Personal communication, August 21, 1998.

59 Bergmann TF, Peterson DH, Lawrence DJ, eds. Chiropractic technique: principles and procedures. New York, NY: Churchill Livingston, 1993.

60 Imrie D, Barbuto, L. The back power program. Toronto, Ontario: Stoddart Publishing, 1988.

CHAPTER 9

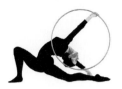

PUBLIC AND MEDICAL ATTITUDES TOWARDS CHIROPRACTIC

A. Public Attitudes

1. **Introduction**. When U.S. state governments, then governments in other countries passed legislation to recognize the new profession of chiropractic early in the 20th century it was solely because of the powerful lobby of satisfied patients. At that time there was strong opposition from the medical profession, and chiropractors themselves had insufficient numbers and status to influence legislators.

   • The key to winning licensure in California in 1922 was the Chiropractic Defenders' League, 28,000 lay persons who had organized huge public rallies and helped to generate more than 2,000 articles in the press in the northern counties alone.[1]

   • When the Danish government introduced funding for chiropractic services into the national health care plan in 1974 it was principally because of a tenacious campaign by the Danish Pro-Chiropractic Association, a large national patient association that had been building public support, lobbying government and funding Gallup polls for over 30 years. (This patient association was founded in January 1925—four months before the Danish Chiropractors' Association—and remains a powerful force today.)

   • When the New Zealand public presented a petition to its government in 1976, seeking funding for chiropractic services under the National Health Care Plan, it was the second largest petition in the country's history and led to the watershed Commission of Inquiry whose report later influenced the acceptance of the chiropractic profession not only in New Zealand but also in Australia and other countries.

   • When the Israeli public, which typically receives its health care through government funded health maintenance organizations (HMOs), demanded government-funded chiropractic services in the mid-1990s HMOs and their affiliated hospitals rapidly provided them.

   The public's attitude towards chiropractic has been basic to the profession's growth and acceptance into mainstream health care. This chapter now looks at surveys of the public's views of the chiropractic profession, utilization rates, satisfaction rates, the role of the media, the role of employers and the new significance of alternative/complementary medicine. What is alternative medicine, why has its growth been so rapid throughout the western world and why is chiropractic seen as being in the forefront of this movement?

   The second section of this chapter reviews medical attitudes towards chiropractic, both those of medical associations and individual physicians. These have had, and continue to have, a significant impact on public attitudes.

2. **Public Surveys**. There is now quite extensive survey research in the U.S. and internationally answering these questions:

   a) *Who uses chiropractic services?* Studies from Australia,[2] Europe,[3] the U.S.[4,5] and Canada[6,7] show that patients are generally representative of the whole adult population and come from all socio-economic groups—all income groups, all occupational groups, all age groups.[2,3,4,5] Children are the one group under-represented. This is what you would expect from a profession whose major fields of practice are back pain and headache.

In some early studies in an era where chiropractic was less known and accepted, such as a U.S. national survey by Saunders Associates in 1954,[8] there were reports of high use by groups with lower income and education. However since the early 1980s studies have consistently reported a trend the other way—patients tending to be from the higher education

... the great majority of patients who use chiropractic services also continue to use medical services—they consult both chiropractic and medical doctors, using each where felt most helpful.

and income groups.[3,4,5] Factors in this shift are ability to pay and make independent choices about health care and the increased acceptance of chiropractic services within the medical and scientific communities.

b) *What is the level of public acceptance?* Wherever the chiropractic profession has become established, general public surveys have reported high levels of acceptance of chiropractic and this has been so for much longer than you might think. For example:

- In the first nationally-based expert survey in the U.S., the one already mentioned by Saunders Associates in 1954 which comprised 658 face-to-face interviews, 39% of American families had at least one member who had received chiropractic care at

some time but 70% favored chiropractic inclusion in prepaid health plans and veterans' hospitals.

- For a good summary of the U.S. surveys during the 1980s see Wardwell.[4] These showed that approximately 3 of 4 individuals responding to independent random telephone surveys in various states had a favorable impression of the chiropractic profession and considered that chiropractic services should be covered by health insurance.

- A 1969 Gallup poll in Denmark showed that 81% of the adult population wanted chiropractors to be recognized by law and funded through the national health plan on a similar basis to medical doctors and dentists.[9]

- A 1990 community survey of 419 adults in the city of Perth, Australia, commissioned by the Health Department of Western Australia reported:[10]

- Approximately 3 out of 4 (72%) agreed that chiropractors "had an important place in the total health system" and this included a substantial majority (69%) of those who had never visited a chiropractor.

- 74% had either used (34%) or would be willing to use (40%) chiropractic services.

- 85% expressed knowledge of what conditions chiropractors treated (principally the spine or back) and 78% knew what methods were used (most commonly manipulation).

In 1995 the chiropractic profession celebrated its centennial, commencing on January 1 with this float in the Rose Parade in Pasadena, California. Famous Americans who stood on the four corners of the float, shown here together before the parade started, are (from left) National League Baseball Hall of Famer, Joe Morgan, country music star Lee Greenwood, 2-time Olympic gold medalist speed skater Cathy Turner, and golfing star Tiger Woods, then-U.S. amateur golf champion. All four are chiropractic patients who donated their time.

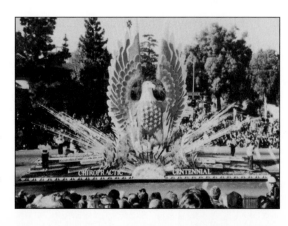

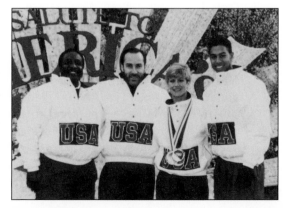

- 89% believed that the cost of chiropractic services should be covered by Medicare, the government's health care plan.

c) *Are patients of chiropractors dissatisfied with medical services?* There are two parts to the answer to this question. Firstly, in general no. Secondly, in relation to the conditions for which they seek chiropractic care—yes.

The surveys show that the great majority of patients who use chiropractic services also continue to use medical services—they consult both chiropractic and medical doctors, using each where felt most helpful. The best study is by Astin from Stanford University.[11] This was a large national survey asking why patients used chiropractic and other forms of alternative health care. One theory being tested was that patients were generally dissatisfied with conventional medical treatment. This was shown not to be true—only 4.4% of those using alternative care expressed strong distrust of or dissatisfaction with medical doctors. Of the 40% of respondents who had used chiropractic or other alternative health care during the previous year, those who said they were "highly satisfied" with medical doctors were as well represented amongst chiropractic patients as those who were dissatisfied with conventional medical care.

There is, however, clear evidence that chiropractic patients are dissatisfied with their medical care for the conditions they take to chiropractors—conditions such as continuing back pain, headache, stress, management of arthritic pain, etc. (See the patient satisfaction studies, and the surveys on the use of alternative and complementary medicine, discussed below in this chapter.)

3. **Utilization Rates**. *United States:* In the U.S. the percentage of the adult population using chiropractic services each year doubled to 10% between 1970 and 1990[12,5] and, even continues to rise though access has become more difficult for many Americans because of restrictive policies in HMOs. National surveys in 1997 by Eisenberg from Harvard[13] and Astin from Stanford[11] report that 11–15% of adult Americans now consult a chiropractor annually.

The exact rate varies by state, and significant factors include the number of chiropractors in practice and levels of third party reimbursement coverage. In 1989 there was a U.S. national ratio of 19 chiropractors per 100,000 population, but this varied from a high in the West and the Plains States (27 per 100,000 and 25 per 100,000 respectively) to a low in New England and the South (14 per 100,000 and 12 per 100,000 respectively.) Federal government forecasting in 1990 pre-

in a recent study from the U.K. medical referrals to chiropractors soared from 2% to 28% of back pain patients when the patient copayment was removed.

dicted a national ratio of 20 chiropractors per 100,000 population in the year 2000, and this now appears accurate.[14] Continued growth in utilization rates can be anticipated. Reasons include:

- the growth in numbers of chiropractors

- the dramatic increase in use of alternative medicine generally—especially among younger adults (ages 18–50)

- the increased integration of chiropractic and medical services now that physicians have accepted that chiropractors have a valuable role in the management of back pain and other spine-related disorders

Canada: In Canada the picture is the same. A 1994/95 national population health survey by Millar of Statistics Canada reports that 11% of Canadians aged 15 and over consulted a chiropractor during the previous 12 months, varying from 17% in the Western and Prairie provinces to approximately 10% in Ontario and Quebec and 3% in Atlantic Canada where there are fewer chiropractors and provincial government health plans do not include coverage for the cost of chiropractic services.[15]

Australia: The Australian survey already mentioned[10] reported that 8% of Western Australian adults had used chiropractic services during the past year in 1990.

Back Pain Patients: What percentage of back pain patients use chiropractic services, and what potential is there for growth of the profession in this area? Studies from the U.S.[16] and Canada[17] report that about 1 in 3 (33%) patients with back pain chooses a chiropractor. Rates in different communities are influenced by how accessible chiropractic services are—restrictions under managed care plans, levels of co-payment from the patient, and the comparative cost and availability of other services. These things are shown dramatically in a recent study from the U.K. where medical referrals to chiropractors soared from 2% to 28% of back pain patients when the patient copayment was removed.[18] (For discussion of this study, see Chapter 8, "Back Pain" page 121.)

Another factor is whether the person making the choice is having a first experience of back pain or has had pain and treatment in the past. The research shows much higher patient satisfaction rates with chiropractic care than with medical care, particularly for back pain. We now look at that evidence.

4. **Patient Satisfaction Rates**. The health care professions and those who manage or pay for health care services are now aware that patient satisfaction is an important measure or "outcome" in health care. This is partly because health care has become a more competitive market with patients more aware of their rights and choices. It is also, however, because patient satisfaction rates are a good measure—in practical terms often the best—of the effectiveness of treatment. Regression analysis of surveys shows that

the effectiveness of care is the single most important factor for patients in assessing their levels of satisfaction.[19]

Chiropractic Services Generally. Satisfaction surveys have consistently shown high satisfaction rates amongst chiropractic patients. One of the first, by Boven in 1976 in Australia was commissioned by the Webb Committee, an Australian federal government *Committee of Inquiry into Chiropractic, Osteopathy, Homeopathy and Naturopathy*.[2] In a representative sample of 627 patients who had seen two or more of a medical practitioner, chiropractor and physiotherapist for a variety of musculoskeletal complaints, satisfaction with chiropractors was markedly higher—51% were very satisfied with chiropractors, as opposed to 16% for physiotherapists and 8% for medical practitioners. At the other end of the scale 12% were not at all satisfied with chiropractors compared with 40% for physiotherapists and 44% for medical practitioner. Fuller results are given in Table 1.

a) The Webb Committee, which comprised three health science academic leaders (2 pharmacologists and a medical physician), drew this conclusion from its review of the Boven et al. study and three other patient surveys it commissioned:

"In summary, chiropractic patients represent a typical cross-section of the adult population, seeking relief for conditions essentially of musculoskeletal origin.... They constitute a significant criticism of the inadequacy of medical therapy for these conditions."[2]

Several U.S. and Canadian studies during the past 10 years have consistently reported satisfaction rates over 75% amongst chiropractic patients. For example, from a 1988 telephone survey of 500 randomly selected households in Connecticut, Wardwell found that 21% had visited a chiropractor. Of those:

- 78% rated the treatment effective or very effective.

- 89% were satisfied or very satisfied with "the amount of personal attention received."

- Only 1 of 2 (51%) had insurance plans that covered chiropractic services.

Table 1 **Degree of Patient Satisfaction for Treatment of Musculoskeletal Complaints**

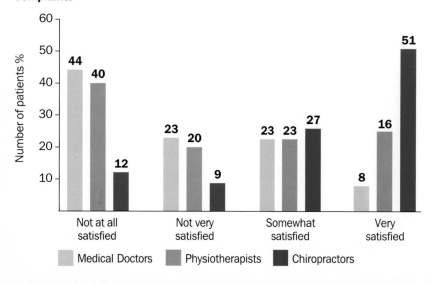

Presumably partly for this reason 1 in 4 (28%) said they were not satisfied with the cost. Three of 4 (72%) said they would visit a chiropractor again "for the same or a similar problem."[20]

b) In a 1990 telephone survey of 693 randomly selected households in New Jersey, Sanchez reports that 29% had visited a chiropractor. Of them:

- 88% were satisfied (23%) or fully satisfied (65%) with the effectiveness of the treatment.

- Nearly all were satisfied or fully satisfied with the chiropractor's professional attitude (97%), competence (93%) and level of attention (96%.)

- Greatest sources of dissatisfaction were the number of visits (29%) and cost (23%). This represented approximately 1 in 4 patients, similar to the Connecticut survey.[21]

c) Sawyer and Kassak in Minnesota studied satisfaction differently—among recent chiropractic patients only and by mailed questionnaire. There was a 70% response rate and, though this is regarded as valid, it may have created some bias in favor of satisfaction. Results included:

- 1 in 2 (47%) considered their health had improved substantially or completely under chiropractic care, whereas only 12% considered that there had been slight (9%) or no (3%) improvement.

- 84% were very satisfied and 97% agreed that they would "recommend their chiropractor to a friend or relative."

- Again, about 1 in 4 (28%) were dissatisfied with cost and inadequate insurance coverage.[19]

d) In 1992 in British Columbia, Canada, Sandhu and Schoner conducted a telephone survey of public attitudes towards health professionals which included a random sample of 150 chiropractic patients from a list provided by the British Columbia Chiropractic Association. Of the 150 past and present patients 83% said they would consult a chiropractor first for their problems once again.[22]

e) In 1998 Decima Research,[17] the polling firm for the Ontario Ministry of Health though commissioned for this study by the Ontario Chiropractic Association, did a random telephone survey of 803 Ontario households with a member "who suffers from back, neck or headache pain for which they have sought treatment from a health practitioner." In other words these were people with experience of the Ontario health care system, where the government plan pays fully for medical services (no direct charge/copayment paid by the patient) but only partly for chiropractic services. (Typically patients have a copayment of $40–$100 for the initial consultation, depending upon what x-rays and other diagnostic tests may be necessary, and a copayment of $20 per treatment visit—the government plan pays approximately $10 per treatment visit.)

In this survey no direct questions were asked on satisfaction. However conclusions on comparative satisfaction with chiropractic and medical care can be drawn from these findings:

Table 2 Treatment Choices by Patients with more than One Episode of Back, Neck and Headache Pain

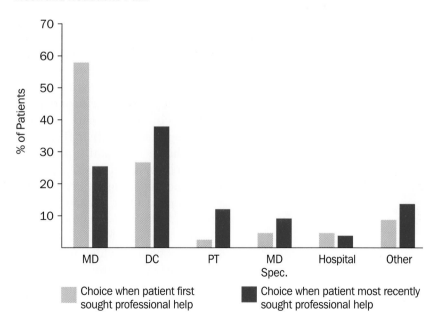

Choice when patient first sought professional help

Choice when patient most recently sought professional help

MD = family physician or general medical practitioner; DC = chiropractor: PT = physical therapist/physiotherapist; MD Spec. = medical specialist; Hospital = hospital emergency department; Other = other or not known (some of the respondents were replying for another member of the household).

- Despite the financial barrier or disincentive to choice of chiropractic care, 1 in 2 (414 or 51%) were users of chiropractic services.

- Over time there was a significant transfer towards chiropractic care illustrated in Table 2. Fifty-eight percent of respondents reported choosing a family physician for their first treatment for back pain and neck pain or headache, versus 25% who chose a chiropractor. For their most recent episode of pain requiring care, only

. . . the media have generally been unhelpful to the chiropractic profession—and other emerging health disciplines such as acupuncture, midwifery and primary care nurse practitioners.

24% chose a family physician, versus 38% who chose a chiropractor.

- Of 142 patients only 1 in 4 (26%) of non-users of chiropractic described their treatment as "very successful." One in 4 (23%) said it was "not very successful" (13%) or "not at all successful" (10%).

  In contrast, 6 in 10 (59%) of recent users of chiropractic rated their treatment very successful, and only 6% said it was not very successful (3%) or not at all successful (3%).

- In this survey there were no direct questions on satisfaction. However conclusions can be drawn from the following significant progression towards chiropractic care. Respondents reported that their first treatment choice was family physician (59%), chiropractor (25%), hospital emergency department (3%), medical specialist (3%), physiotherapist (2%) and other/do not know (8%). This compares with the most recent treatment choice, which was family physician (24%), chiropractor (38%), hospital emergency department (2%), medical specialist (9%), physiotherapist (11%) and other/do not know (12%).

f) A 1997 survey by the New Zealand Consumer Institute, asking 8,007 of its members about their use of alternative therapies, found that chiropractic, herbal medicine and homeopathy were the most widely used therapies. The Consumer Institute reported, however, that "of these only chiropractic had a high satisfaction rating (74%)."[23]

Back Pain. The above studies are relevant to back pain also. This is because 65-70% of all chiropractic patients have back pain and therefore the majority of patients in the studies will have been reporting satisfaction with chiropractic treatment for back pain.

However there are satisfaction surveys specifically relating to back pain patients. The studies to 1993 are reviewed in the *Manga Report*.[24] They are supported by more recent studies.[16,17,19] The most thorough comparative study dealt with 457 back pain patients at a Washington HMO who had visited either family physicians (215 patients) or chiropractors (242). This looked at specific causes of satisfaction or dissatisfaction and found:

a) The percentage of chiropractic patients who were "very satisfied" with the care they received for low-back pain was 3 times that of patients of family physicians (66% versus 22%).

b) Common reasons for higher satisfaction care included:

   - More information received about the back problems, including the cause of pain, recovery from pain, content of care and instructions on exercise, posture and lifting.

   - The amount of time the chiropractor spent listening to their description of the pain.

   - The chiropractor's belief that the pain was real and expression of concern.

   - Doctor confidence in the diagnosis and effectiveness of treatment.[25]

5. **Role of the Media**: Public attitudes are obviously strongly influenced by the media, which have generally been unhelpful to the chiropractic profession—and other emerging health disciplines such as acupuncture, dental hygiene, homeopathy, massage therapy, midwifery and primary care and specialized nurse practitioners. A significant

cause is that, in the area of health, Associated Press, Reuters, major daily newspapers, and radio/television networks are hard-wired to medical sources which set the tone for most of their material on chiropractic and other health professions. To illustrate this:

a) The only good news about chiropractic that becomes a "story" in the mass media is news filtered through a medical source. Until the mid-1980s this never happened. At that point major collaborative research between the chiropractic and medical professions became possible and this (examples of which are the 1990 Meade trial on back pain in the U.K. funded by the Medical Research Council,[26] the 1991 RAND Report on manipulation in the U.S.[27] and the 1994 U.S. government-sponsored back pain guide-

lines)[28] finally led to positive research-based stories on the effectiveness of chiropractic in the mass media.

However exciting research discoveries from purely chiropractic researchers have always gone, and continue to go, unnoticed in the media. A good example is the evidence during the 1990s that headache originating in the cervical spine is as common as migraine, is often medically misdiagnosed as migraine or tension headache and responds better to chiropractic manipulation than tradi-

The public is inundated with media stories that reinforce the scientific basis and high quality of medical education. Today chiropractic educational standards and licensing exams are of similar quality, but that story is never told.

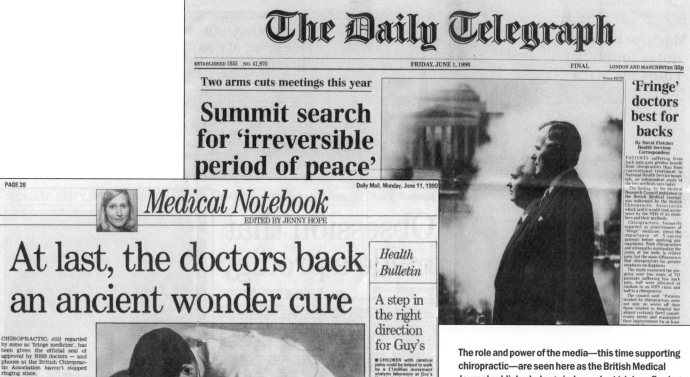

The role and power of the media—this time supporting chiropractic—are seen here as the British Medical Journal published a large independent trial confirming that chiropractic treatment was more effective than conventional medical services for adults with acute and chronic low-back pain. On the same day the British national newspaper *The Daily Telegraph* gave this news front-page treatment alongside the Bush/Gorbachev Summit. Ten days later another British national paper, *The Daily Mail*, reports: "Chiropractic, still regarded by some as 'fringe medicine', has been given the official seal of approval by NHS doctors—and phones at the British Chiropractic Association haven't stopped ringing since."

tional medical treatments. (For references to this research, see Chapter 6, page 75.)

b) On the other hand purely medical sources have little difficulty generating mass media comment on presumed shortcomings in the effectiveness and safety of chiropractic care. Two recent examples are:

- In 1994, Carlini, a California neurologist, reported a survey of his colleagues on the frequency of stroke following chiropractic manipulation.[29] Firstly it had little scientific validity—it was a simple retrospective survey asking neurologists to estimate their experience, and there was an unacceptably low response rate (36%.) Secondly the survey showed nothing new—it confirmed existing evidence of a risk rate of 1 per 500,000 manipulations. Thirdly Carlini expressly acknowledged that "the safety of cervical chiropractic treatments is not being challenged by these findings" and that "most interventions by physicians have a higher complication rate."

  However Carlini was from the Stanford Stroke Center, his survey was done in collaboration with the American Academy of Neurology and its preliminary results were presented at a large medical meeting sponsored by the American Heart Association. During the following days, an Associated Press item published in newspapers throughout North America and Europe was headlined *Twist of the Neck can Cause Stroke Warn Doctors*. In graphic language it gave the impression that chiropractic manipulation was a common and dangerous cause of stroke and it quoted the off-the-cuff, unsupported comment of one neurologist that "every neurologist in this room has seen 2 or 3 people who have suffered (stroke) after chiropractic manipulation."

  (In contrast, you may be interested to know that there was no publicity given to much more thorough research published at the same time in the journal *Neurology*, research

which looked at stroke referrals in four major hospitals in the U.S. and Germany and found that avoidable strokes from incorrect patient neck positioning by anesthesiologists during general anesthesia was a much more common problem.[30])

- In 1998 a Washington HMO trial of two forms of chiropractic and physical therapy management of patients with low-back pain showed patients in both treatment groups doing significantly better than control group patients after four weeks but not on long term follow-up. Patients were highly satisfied with care. Average total diagnostic and treatment costs per chiropractic patient were $230.00, less than the cost of a single MRI or CT scan of the type routinely ordered by medical doctors for back pain patients. Again, this study reported nothing new.

  However the trial was published in the Massachusetts Medical Society's *New England Journal of Medicine*[31] which asked whether the benefits were worth the cost. Established news links between medical sources and news services led to a quite astounding international barrage of negative articles from Texas to Tokyo under titles such as *Chiropractic Care Blasted*.[32] (Incidentally, the medical authors of the study have been criticized for an obviously flawed analysis of costs.[33] Chiropractic patients experienced less disability during the 12 months following treatment, and the total cost of chiropractic care may have been more than recovered by reduced disability/compensation costs—however that data was not provided.)

c) Consider the field of education. The public is inundated with media stories and programs that reinforce the scientific basis and high quality of medical education. Today chiropractic educational standards and licensing exams are of similar quality (see Chapter 4, "Education and Licensure") but that story is never told. Focus testing shows that the public has a poor understanding of the length and quality of chiropractic education. The chiropractic profession has actually had to buy advertising space to begin to address this problem.

Consumers' Associations. Another major past source of bad press for the chiropractic profession has been medical critics acting under the guise and apparent credibility of consumer organizations. Three long-term foes of this type, already mentioned in Chapter 1, are Dr. Stephen Barrett, advisor to the U.S. Consumers' Union, Dr. William Jarvis, founder and President of the National Council Against Health Fraud Inc., and Dr. Murray Katz, advisor to the Consumers' Association of Canada.

Commentators have observed, with good reason, that a consumers' association is excellent for rating products, because it can commission and fund the relatively short-term and inexpensive research required. However, it has a less clear role in judging professional services. Surveys of public attitudes may be possible, but in reporting on the education, qualifications and effectiveness of health professionals, it is simply reliant on the views of the consultants it chooses. Medical consultants will likely be unreliable in judging other competing professions.

The More Educated Periodicals. In this sector the chiropractic profession has had significant help from the media. Moore[34] analyzes the content and tone of all articles on chiropractic appearing in the U.S. popular periodical press (defined as publications intended for a general educated audience and achieving widespread circulation) from four articles in *Harper's Weekly* in 1915 with titles like "Mail Order Miracle Men" through to articles in the *Atlantic, Runners' World* and *Prevention* in 1988/89. The articles are graded extremely negative, negative, neutral, positive, and extremely positive. Almost all articles, except those by chiropractors, were extremely negative through to the mid-1970s. At that time, interestingly, there was a dramatic swing and most articles thereafter have been positive or extremely positive. Reasons will have included the strong development in chi-

ropractic education, practice standards and licensure during the 1960s and 1970s.

Conclusion: To conclude, there are instances of fraudulent behavior and grossly unprofessional claims by some chiropractors from time to time and it is obviously appropriate for the media, as in two investigative reports by the television program *20/20* in the 1990s, to expose and comment on this behavior. However, the chiropractic profession has a just complaint that its achieve-

... a consumers' association is excellent for rating products ... it has a less clear role in judging professional services. Surveys reporting on the education, qualifications and effectiveness of health professionals are simply reliant on the views of the consultants it chooses.

ments in education, practice, research and its overall contribution to health, have not been presented by the media in an unbiased and fair manner. Reporters receiving information on chiropractic from a medical source, directly or indirectly through a service such as Associated Press, frequently fail to take the fundamental first step of fair journalism of consulting a chiropractic source for comment. In North America such sources include:

- *Professional associations.* National associations in the U.S. (American Chiropractic Association, Arlington VA, tel: 703-276-8800, International Chiropractors' Association, Arlington VA, tel: 703-528-5000) and in Canada (Canadian Chiropractic Association, Toronto, Ontario, tel: 416-781-5656).

- *Educational authorities.* In the U.S. the Council on Chiropractic Education, Scottsdale AZ, tel: 602-443-8877 and the Association of Chiropractic Colleges, Bethesda, MD, tel: 301-652-5066, and in Canada, the Canadian Council on Chiropractic Education, Richmond, British Columbia, tel: 604-278-3505, or the Canadian Memorial Chiropractic

College, Toronto, Ontario, tel: 416-482-2340.

- *Licensing organizations.* In the U.S. the Federation of Chiropractic Licensing Boards, Greely CO, tel: 970-356-3500 and in Canada the Canadian Federation of Chiropractic Regulatory Boards, Toronto, Ontario, tel: 416-486-0005.

(For further details on these and other organizations see Chapter 3, "Current Status of the Profession" page 128.)

Savings of this magnitude are certain to mean that the corporate world will have a much greater say in shaping general attitudes to chiropractic services in the years immediately ahead.

6. **Role of Business**: This has been surprisingly small, given that disability from back pain is by far the greatest cause of employer health care and compensation costs, and that there has now been good evidence since the mid-1980s that the integration of chiropractic and medical services leads to major cost savings and much higher patient satisfaction rates.

One reason why business has been slow to act may be the fact that many major corporations have dealt with different carriers for employee benefits, workers' compensation and disability insurances. This means they have not had the data linking health care and disability costs. There are many signs that things are about to change because:

- There is now clear evidence from interdisciplinary clinical guidelines and the reports of health economists on the appropriate management of back pain and the substantial cost savings this can bring. These give skilled manipulation and the chiropractic profession a major role. In Canada Manga and Angus, University of Ottawa health economists, predict that a doubling in the number of musculoskeletal pain patients consulting a chiropractor first would lead to savings of $1.85 billion per annum in disability costs in the province of Ontario (population 8 million).[24]

- Corporations that have remodelled their occupational health strategies on the

basis of this new evidence report significant savings. These range from large employers such as the Rover Group[35] to small employers such as two U.K. companies with 750 employees which realized 18% savings in the first year and 40% savings in the second year in net disability costs when they subsidized a plan whereby employees complaining of neck/arm or back/leg pain were initially referred for chiropractic treatment during 1994/95.[36]

- After training 20,000 flight attendants with the *BACKSAFE* prevention program designed and led by chiropractors, United Airlines experienced a 63% reduction in back and neck injuries. (This was from the fourth quarter of 1996, when *BACKSAFE* was initiated, to the first quarter of 1998. For comment on other corporate prevention programs and savings, see page 89.)

- Savings of this magnitude, usually flowing from a combination of prevention programs, appropriate care, workplace redesign and improved return to work programs, are certain to mean that the corporate world will have a much greater say in shaping general attitudes to chiropractic services in the years immediately ahead. (For more on cost-effectiveness see Chapter 8, "Back Pain," Section C, pages 118–120.)

7. **Complementary and Alternative Medicine (CAM)**: A major shift in societal attitudes to health in Europe, North America and the industrialized world during the 1990s has been the greatly increased acceptance and use of complementary or alternative medicine (CAM)—approaches such as chiropractic, acupuncture, homeopathy, herbal medicine—and the desire of patients to integrate CAM and medical care, using each where found most safe and effective. We now look at:

- the definition of CAM
- to what extent it is now used by the public, and why
- acknowledgement by the medical profession that this use reflects true public needs and is here to stay

- how influential chiropractic is in the CAM movement, and

- the significance of this on public attitudes towards the profession.

(Ironically the chiropractic profession sees itself as an independent licensed profession rather than *complementary* or *alternative* or *medicine*. However, as will be seen, the medical profession [and thus health authorities and thus the public] identifies chiropractic as the leading and most developed example of a CAM discipline.)

a) *Definition of CAM.* There is no agreed terminology or definition. *Alternative medicine* is the preferred term in the U.S., *complementary medicine* in the U.K. The word *alternative* means *in place of* while the word *complementary* means *alongside and in conjunction with* and, as the British Medical Association (BMA) has acknowledged, this means that chiropractic is both complementary and alternative to medical treatment.[37]

The most widely accepted definition in the U.S. is that used by Eisenberg from Harvard, namely that CAMs are "medical interventions not taught widely at U.S. medical schools or generally available at U.S. hospitals." In their 1991[5] and 1997[12] national telephone surveys, respondents were given these 16 examples of CAM—relaxation techniques, chiropractic, massage, imagery, spiritual healing, commercial weight-loss programs, lifestyle, diets (e.g. macrobiotics), herbal medicine, mega vitamin therapy, self-help groups, energy healing, biofeedback, hypnosis, homeopathy, acupuncture and folk remedies.

In the U.K. the BMA's definition of CAM is "those forms of treatment which are not widely used by the orthodox health care professions, and the skills of which are not taught as part of the undergraduate curriculum of orthodox medical and paramedical health care courses."[37] The BMA regards acupuncture, chiropractic, herbalism, homeopathy and osteopathy as the five most developed CAM disciplines and those with "the potential for greatest use alongside orthodox medical care."

Elsewhere the BMA acknowledges that CAM therapies are grouped together "not because of any commonality of principle or practice but because they stand outside the parameters of that health care which is standardly available on the National Health Service." Accordingly the essence of CAM is that it is health care methods that have not generally been taught in the core curriculum of medical schools.

b) *How Widespread is the Use of CAM?* Acceptance and use are now extremely

The British Medical Association regards acupuncture, chiropractic, herbalism, homeopathy and osteopathy as the five most developed CAM disciplines and those with "the potential for greatest use alongside orthodox medical care."

widespread, with nearly 1 in 2 persons using CAM during the past 12 months in Australia,[38] Canada,[39] the United States[5] and Europe.[40] As many as 2 out of 3 medical patients are also using CAM for various chronic pain syndromes and diseases,[5,41] and the great majority of general medical practitioners are now referring patients for CAM in Europe[42] and North America.[43,44]

c) *Why Do People Use CAM?* This question has been examined most thoroughly in Europe by Furnham[45] and in the U.S. by Astin.[10] They are in agreement and their findings are confirmed by a 1997 national poll in Canada.[16] In summary:

i) The two dominant factors for CAM users are dissatisfaction with medical care for their current complaint (the push factor—pushing them towards CAM) and belief in the effectiveness of the CAM approach (the pull factor—attracting them to CAM).

ii) The second factor is actually the dominant one. CAM users have greater awareness of physiology and health than medical patients, have more self-aware and ecologically aware lifestyles and have greater belief that treatment should concentrate on the whole person. They are pulled towards CAM because it is "more natural, effective, relaxing, sensible and one can take an active part in it."

iii) However CAM users do not reject orthodox medicine altogether and do not have "noticeably different health belief models compared with similar patients who are exclusive users of orthodox medicine." None of the simple hypotheses for why people use CAM are true—for example that they are turned off orthodox medicine, that they have a pronounced philosophy or lifestyle that fits CAM

"When all is said and done, what works will no longer be called mainstream or complementary—it will just be called good medicine." *–Marc Micozzi, MD, PhD*

or that they have a particular neurotic or psychosomatic profile. The studies show that CAM patients are a normal cross-section of the population shopping for health. Where various forms of CAM are available they will likely use more than one—these health shoppers will use orthodox medicine for broken bones, chiro-

practic and acupuncture for back pain and headache and homeopathy for allergies.

Consumer and medical commentators agree. In one of the most powerful consumer books, *Reclaiming Our Health* by John Robbins,[46] whose first book was *Diet for a New America*, the author:

- Analyzes the basis of the current rise of CAM in the United States. Robbins links it to dissatisfaction with the "medicalization of life" arising from a combination of the following factors—ignoring the inherent powers of the body; removing personal control of health, and freedom of choice; and doing this in many circumstances where "dominator medicine" is less effective than CAM and has unacceptable costs, risks and side effects.

  He gives many powerful examples, including the medicalization of childbirth and menopause and the quite ruthless suppression of natural therapies for cancer.

- Concludes that the public does not want to turn its back on orthodox medicine but that it wants self-determination in health care; the medical doctor as collaborator not dictator; and an end to the medical monopoly and the creation of "a medical system that includes the alternative and drugless modes of healing in true partnership."

Also in the U.S. Wayne Jonas, MD, Past Director of the Center for Alternative Medicine, National Institutes of Health, writing an editorial in a November 1998 issue of *The Journal of the American Medical Association* which was fully devoted to CAM, advises medical doctors that "alternative medicine is here to stay" because it "reflects changing needs and values in modern society in general."[47]

d) *How Big is Chiropractic in CAM?* In the U.S. Eisenberg national survey (1998)[12] reports:

- 4 in 10 Americans used at least one alternative therapy in 1997. For adults aged 35–49 years, 1 of every 2 persons used CAM.

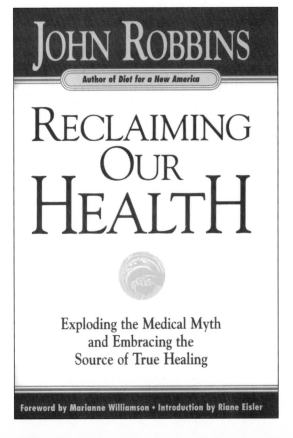

Reclaiming Our Health, ISBN 0-915811-69-3, H. J. Kramer Inc., Tiburon, CA. "In this wonderful new book John Robbins meticulously documents how and why the factors associated with true healing are often missing from the so-called health care systems of our country, and then gives us some very uplifting and practical solutions to this dilemma." Christiane Northrup, MD, Assistant Clinical Professor, Obstetrics and Gynecology, University of Vermont, College of Medicine, author of *Women's Bodies, Women's Wisdom*.

JOHN ROBBINS

Author of *Diet for a New America*

RECLAIMING OUR HEALTH

Exploding the Medical Myth and Embracing the Source of True Healing

Foreword by Marianne Williamson • Introduction by Riane Eisler

- 11% of the adult population used chiropractic care, which is the single most used form of CAM.

- Total annual visits for CAM increased by 47% between 1990 and 1997 to 629 million, which exceeded total visits to all U.S. primary care physicians by 243 million.

- Annual expenditures rose by 45% exclusive of inflation over the same period. They were conservatively estimated at $21.2 billion, $12.2 billion of this was paid out-of-pocket, and this exceeded out-of-pocket expenditure for all U.S. hospitalizations.

Another U.S. national survey at approximately the same time by Astin from the Stanford University School of Medicine,[10] places chiropractic utilization slightly higher —the four top treatment categories in CAM were chiropractic (15.7%), lifestyle/diet (8%), exercise/movement (7.2%) and relaxation (6.9%.) Accordingly chiropractic services were used twice as much as any other form of CAM. Astin reports that chiropractors were commonly used for various chronic pain and anxiety syndromes and provided "close to 50% of all alternative treatments used for headaches."

In Canada chiropractic services are even more dominant within CAM. A 1994/95 survey by Statistics Canada[14] and a 1997 survey by CTV/Angus Reid[39] report that chiropractic services are used annually by about 15% of the adult population and are used three times more commonly than the next most popular forms of CAM—herbology, acupuncture and homeopathy.

e) *Conclusion:* Current public acceptance and use of CAM in general have led to more public and medical knowledge and acceptance of chiropractic specifically. Medical leaders, such as Dr. Marc Micozzi of Philadelphia in the statement which opens the next section, agree that, as various forms of complementary and alternative care such as chiropractic manipulation become more fully integrated into health care services, they will no longer be regarded as CAM but simply as good health care.

B. Medical Attitudes

1. Introduction:

"The Agency for Health Care Policy and Research (AHCPR) recently made history when it concluded that spinal manipulative therapy is the most effective and cost-effective treatment for acute low-back pain. . . . One might conclude that for acute low-back pain not caused by fracture, tumor, infection, or the cauda equina syndrome, spinal manipulation is the treatment of choice.

"Because acute low-back pain is the most prevalent ailment and most frequent cause of disability for persons younger than 45 years of age in the United States, adherence to these practice guidelines could substantially increase the numbers of patients referred for spinal manipulation. Chiropractors provide 94% of spinal manipulation.

"As physicians are becoming increasingly willing and able to justify referral for complementary care . . . we must foster the development of training, research and clinical protocols to support integration . . . in a way that promotes favorable clinical outcomes.

"Alternative medicine can benefit from the kind of support from which mainstream medicine has benefited over the years. When all is said and done, what works will no longer be called mainstream or complementary—it will just be called good medicine."

Marc Micozzi, MD, PhD,
College of Physicians of Philadelphia
Annals of Internal Medicine 1998.[48]

The above quote, from an eminent U.S. physician in the official journal of the American College of Physicians, illustrates how much medical attitudes to chiropractic have changed over the past 20 years. It appears in an editorial commenting on a study on the appropriateness of chiropractic care appearing in the same issue of the *Annals*. In the early 1980s the American College of Physicians was one of several defendants in *Wilk* v *American Medical Association*, a class action brought by the chiropractic profession against a cartel of medical associations, and it was more likely that Jesse Helms would speak in honor of Fidel Castro than the

Annals would print an endorsement of the chiropractic profession. Much has changed.

Medical attitudes towards chiropractic, and vice versa, have been and continue to be of fundamental significance to public attitudes towards chiropractic and the development of the profession. That is why they are now reviewed. Much of the content of previous chapters is relevant including:

- The overall reasons for conflict in the past and greater cooperation today. (Chapter 2, "Chiropractic History," Section C, E and F.)

- The common chiropractic and medical approach to management of back pain patients today, and the interdisciplinary research and clinical guidelines that have produced this agreement. (Chapter 8, "Back Pain," Section C and D, 2–6.)

- The collaboration of chiropractic and medical authors in producing many texts and scientific journals. (Chapter 3, "Current Status of the Profession," Section E.)

2. **Medical Associations**: These, like chiropractic associations, are trade organizations whose fundamental mission is to protect the profession and economic interests of their members. In the past medical associations have been ruthless in trying to eliminate the chiropractic profession as a competitor. A prime tactic, used successfully for many years by the American Medical Association (AMA) and affiliated medical organizations, was to portray the chiropractic profession as an unscientific cult, at the same time working to undermine chiropractic education and research and to prevent AMA members from working with chiropractors in education, research and practice. It took full battle in protracted litigation, the *Wilk* case, to begin to redress that misinformation campaign. (See Chapter 2, "Chiropractic History," page 14.)

Medical associations in North America continue covert action against the chiropractic profession, particularly at the cutting edge of access to services. For example, working with members and allies in the U.S. administration and Blue Cross/Blue Shield, U.S. medical associations have engineered policy and now regulations producing a remarkable result under Medicare. As of December 1998 the Health Care Financing Authority (HCFA) has provided the legal opinion that chiropractic services under Medicare, defined as "manual manipulation of the spine to correct a subluxation," services which nobody disputes are defined in chiropractic language and were negotiated by the American Chiropractic Association and introduced to give seniors access to chiropractic services, may be provided by medical and osteopathic doctors when given in HMOs. Armed with this HCFA interpretation, Blue Cross of California has dropped coverage of chiropractic services under its Senior Secure Plan in the Northern California region, its HMO plan for seniors. The ACA has filed a lawsuit against the U.S. government.

However North American medical associations need to be much more careful about their public stances on chiropractic. Former rulings against cooperation with the chiropractic profession are gone, individual physicians are free to cooperate with chiropractors and generally do because of their patients' best interests and patient demand, and the attack of organized medicine on chiropractic is much weakened. This is particularly so in bodies with public (lay) representation such as medical licensing boards.

Therefore, for example, the College of Physicians and Surgeons of Ontario (CPSO), Canada's largest self-regulatory board for physicians but one with 9 public members, produced policy expressly authorizing physicians to refer patients to chiropractors when it was obliged through public pressure to develop policy on complementary and alternative medicine in 1997. This new policy was made both on the basis of patient freedom of choice and the acknowledgement that chiropractic was a "complementary discipline of healing" that had "established a historical and respected role in healing and required arduous training and evaluation."[49]

Medical associations in many other countries remain open opponents of the chiropractic profession. Refreshing examples of cooperation are found in the U.K. The British Medical Association (BMA) has been openly supportive of the development and regulation of chiropractic services since the 1993 publication of its study into complementary medicine, on the grounds that chiropractic is an established discipline and many BMA members wish to refer patients for chiropractic care.[37] The U.K. Royal College of General Practitioners has worked co-operatively with the British Chiropractic Association in the development of clinical practice guidelines for the same reason.

There is also cooperation at the international level, where principle seems to triumph over practical politics more easily. The World Federation of Neurology and the World Federation of Public Health Associations, together with the International Council of Nurses all actively supported the World Federation of Chiropractic during its 1997 admission into official relations with the World Health Organization and membership of the Council of International Organizations of Medical Sciences—the WHO affiliate representing the international organizations for various medical specialties and other health professionals. As the World Federation of Neurology observed in its letter of support "the relationship between the medical and chiropractic professions worldwide has become increasingly one of mutual respect and collaboration."[50]

3. **Physicians in Practice**: In Dallas, the Texas Back Institute, one of the most sophisticated surgical and conservative spinal care facilities in the U.S., has four chiropractors on staff and one is a partner. There are chiropractors on staff at the Asaf Harofeh Hospital in Tel Aviv, Israel; at Kimberley Hospital, Kimberly, South Africa; and at hundreds of other hospitals and multidisciplinary spinal care centers throughout the world. Medical surveys of family physicians in the U.S. and Canada show that a majority of physicians are either referring patients to chiropractors,[51] or would like to.[52] In short, we are currently in an era in which medical doctors are being told in their own literature and by patients that chiropractic services have a valuable role within the health care system and doctors are generally accepting that message.

In the U.S. the public's now widespread and established demand for chiropractic and other complementary and alternative medicine (CAM), discussed earlier in this chapter (pages 134–137), means that prominent medical centers that would not have considered having chiropractic services a few years

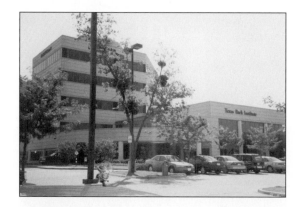

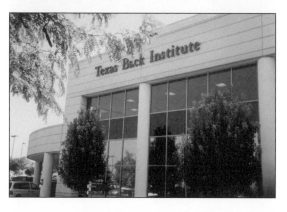

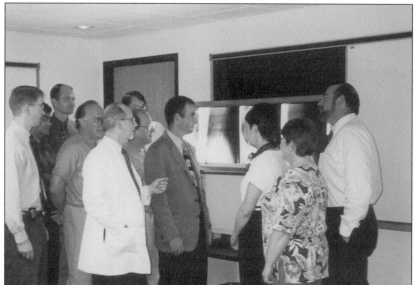

At the Texas Back Institute in Dallas, which offers a full range of conservative and surgical treatments in one of the most sophisticated back-care facilities in the U.S., one of the four staff chiropractors Dr. John Triano presents a case to other staff physicians, surgeons and physical therapists during the regular interdisciplinary review of interesting cases on weekly rounds.

ago are now incorporating them. An example is New York City's Beth Israel Medial Center, a major clinical and academic medical center affiliated with three other medical schools and hospitals. In an interview published in early 1999, Dr. Woodson Merrell explained:

- The future of good and effective primary care in America is "integrated medicine," combining medical care with chiropractic, acupuncture, homeopathy and other established forms of complementary medicine.

- This was not simply his view, or the attitude of a few enthusiasts on staff, but was broadly accepted at every level at the Beth Israel Medical Center. "When I went to talk to the chairs of the other departments virtually no chair was opposed to the idea of the (integrated medicine) center whereas three years ago these people would have been apoplectic, jumping over themselves to get

me out of the room . . . there's been a radical shift."

- The move to integrated medicine, including chiropractic services, was not an entrepreneurial venture—Beth Israel is an academic center backed by a number of hospitals and medical schools which is going to combine clinical services and ongoing research. Following Dr. Merrell's interview, various prominent medical centers around the U.S., including centers at Harvard and Stanford, are moving to the same integrated model.[53]

Factors that have kept the medical and chiropractic professions apart in the past but are leading to a future of integration and co-operation are reviewed in Chapter 2, "Chiropractic History" and Chapter 8, "Back Pain" —especially Section C.) However there are still a number of factors restricting this new partnership between medicine and chiropractic and inter-referral of patients, and these may be summarized as follows:

At the Spine and Rehabilitation Center in Austin, Texas, neurosurgeon Dr. Alan Williams (left) and chiropractor Dr. Bill Defoyd review imaging studies at their multidisciplinary facility.

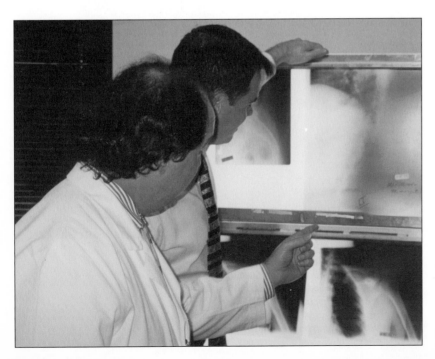

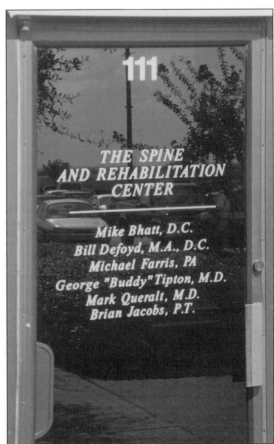

a) *The continuing unprofessional claims of some chiropractors with respect to scope of practice.* A 1990 survey of family physicians in Ontario, Canada showed that 62% were referring patients to chiropractors, almost exclusively for musculoskeletal pain, but that by far the greatest concern of all physicians—including 83% of those who were "referring patients or open to referral"—was the scope of chiropractic practice and claims by chiropractors to be able to treat "organic diseases."[50] (Interestingly, data from two surveys of chiropractic practice in Ontario at the time of the above physician survey showed that 96% of chiropractic practice was for patients with musculoskeletal problems.[11,51] So the basis for concern over scope of practice was not strong.)

This historic medical concern has two aspects. One is a lack of understanding of the possible, and for some patients fundamentally important, link between neuromusculoskeletal dysfunction and a wide range of conditions. (See Chapter 5, "Principles and Goals of Chiropractic," and Chapter 6, "Scope of Practice.")

However a second aspect is the continuing irresponsible claims on scope of practice by some chiropractors. All professions have a fringe element. But this fringe element is particularly damaging to the chiropractic profession because of its history, or, in the language of sociology, because of the chiropractic profession's lack of cultural authority compared with more established professions.

b) *A Lack of Understanding of Chiropractic Education and Practice.* Most medical doctors received no introduction to chiropractic and other complementary health care disciplines at medical school and have had no formal or traditional methods of establishing linkages with chiropractors in their communities.

Surveys during the past 10 years consistently show that physicians want more opportunities to learn about chiropractic services. Until recently that has happened by informal methods such as occasional presentations by chiropractors on medical continuing education programs and during hospital rounds, and articles on chiropractic by medical and chiropractic authors in the medical literature.

Since the mid-1980s interdisciplinary societies such as the American Back Society (2647 East 14th Street, Suite 401, Oakland CA, 94601 USA, tel: 510-536-9929, fax: 510-536-1812, email: ambasoc@aol.com, website: www.americanbacksoc.org) and the North American Cervicogenic Headache Society (York Mills Centre, 16 York Mills Road, Unit 125, Box 129, North York, Ontario M2P 2E5, Canada, tel: 416-512-6407, fax: 416-512-6375, email: reception@rothbart.com) have given physicians opportunities to meet professionally with chiropractors.

More formal methods of education have emerged in the past few years. Eisenberg has recently reported that over 60% of medical schools in the U.S., including Harvard and other Ivy League schools, now have introductory courses on complementary medicine including chiropractic, both for medical students and in continuing education programs for practicing physicians.

In the U.K. the Royal College of General Practitioners (RCGP) has not only developed formal clinical guidelines for the management of patients with back pain in a process that included representatives of the British Chiropractic Association, but currently has an interdisciplinary team led by chiropractor Alan Breen, DC, PhD, from the Anglo-European College of Chiropractic in Bournemouth, that is developing a package of audit materials that will be sent to every general practitioner. This material, which is designed to encourage physicians to comply with the RCGP's clinical guidelines, will include information on chiropractic and the importance of skilled manipulation, which is one of the first options for treatment recommended for most back pain patients.

c) *Lack of a Referral Network*: This is a related problem. Today most family physicians may be willing to refer patients to a chiropractor but how does one find "a good chiropractor"? Chiropractors have

Signage from clinics throughout North America offering
integrated chiropractic and
medical services.

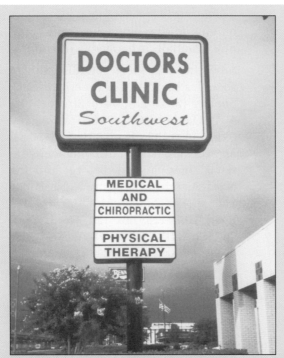

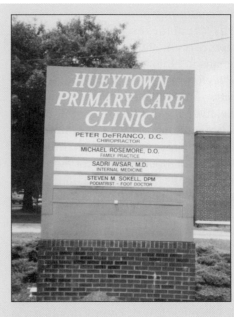

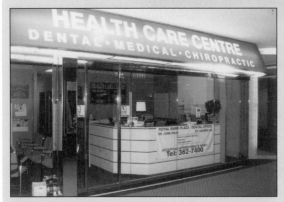

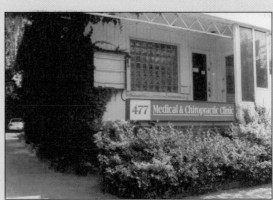

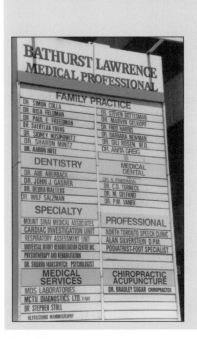

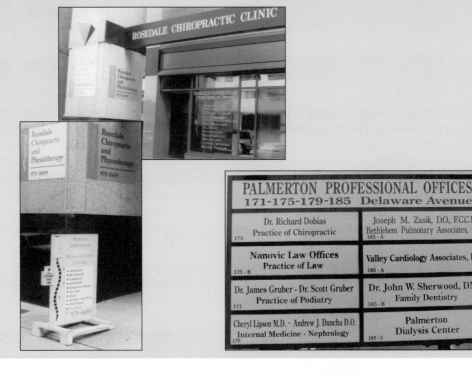

traditionally been in private practice, typically in a home/office setting remote from medical centers. As already indicated, the marketplace is solving this problem naturally. The 1990 survey of family physicians in Canada showed that 62% were referring patients but that the referral rate was 100% for those who had a chiropractor in or adjacent to their medical center or office building.

d) *Structural and Financial Access Difficulties:* Medical concerns about the education and beliefs of chiropractors are an issue as explained above, but structural and financial barriers to cooperation are a more important issue for physicians and patients today:

- *Structural.* Many physicians would like access to chiropractic services but health maintenance organizations (HMOs), other managed care plans, regional health authorities or patient employee benefits plans under which they work do not include these services.

- *Financial.* Of all issues being discussed, this is the key barrier today. Physicians who accept that certain patients would receive best results under chiropractic care are reluctant to recommend a chiropractor for many of these patients when there is a "free" funded alternative—and many patients want to start with the "free" service too. This is well illustrated by the U.K. study referred to in Chapter 8, "Back Pain" (para 9, page 121)—in a pilot project involving 11 GP practices the referral rate to chiropractors for back pain patients went from 2% to 28%, and the overall referral rate for skilled manipulation from 2% to 53% (28% chiropractors, 25% osteopaths), when the Wiltshire Health Authority provided funding for "manipulation services" in accordance with the Royal College of General Practitioners' back pain guidelines.

In the U.S. Shekelle has shown that out-of-pocket costs to the patient are a much greater barrier to access to chiropractic services than general medical care, out-patient medical care or dental care.

In technical language, chiropractic remains very "cost-sensitive." Where the patient co-payment is 25% of the fee or greater, utilization of chiropractic services falls by approximately 50%. When patients have similar co-payments for chiropractic and medical care, and are then given free medical care, utilization of fee-for-service chiropractic care falls by 80%.[54]

4. **Physicians in Education and Research**. The fields of education and research attract health professionals of like mind and similar interests, whether they are physicians, chiropractors or other. Birds of a feather flock together. Not surprisingly, therefore, the new collaboration between medicine and chiropractic was first built largely by practitioners who were also active leaders in continuing education and research.

The acknowledged medical leaders in research into the management of back pain—people such as Dr. Richard Deyo (University of Washington), Dr. Norton Hadler (University of North Carolina, Chapel Hill), Dr. Vert Mooney (University of California at San Diego, Past-President, International Society for the Study of the Lumbar Spine [ISSLS]), Dr. Jim Weinstein (University of Iowa and Editor, *Spine*) and Dr. Arthur White (San Francisco Spine Institute) in the U.S., Dr. William Kirkaldy-Willis in Canada, Dr. Gordon Waddell in the U.K., Dr. Bjorn Rydevik in Sweden, Dr. Karel Lewit in the Czech Republic, and Dr. Jivi Dvorak in Switzerland—have all spoken at chiropractic research conferences and encouraged collaborative research and practice. As a few brief examples:

- Speaking on the importance of collaborative chiropractic and medical research at the Chiropractic Centennial Conference in Washington, DC, in July 1995 Dr. Jim Weinstein, editor of the leading journal *Spine* and an orthopedic surgeon, said:

"New alliances must be formed in order to advance those whom we treat . . . Collaborative research is not the future, it is now. Together we must move forward to meet the new challenges of education, research and patient care . . . it is our challenge of the next century to find the level ground to form collaborative relationships that seek to find answers on many different planes and bring forward a revolution in medicine."[55]

• At the same meeting Dr. Arthur White, also an orthopedic surgeon and speaking from his experience of integrating chiropractic services in California managed care settings, referred to the new U.S. government-sponsored guidelines acknowledging the valuable role of manipulation for patients with acute low-back pain and concluded:

"The new managed care system directs patient to the least expensive professional who can get the job done most efficiently and accurately. With minimal redirection the chiropractor is the ideal professional to diagnose and treat the early phases of spinal problems, and can easily triage (*i.e. diagnose and refer*) patients to the most appropriate chronic health care providers . . . We all need to prepare for the 21st century . . . There are some definite trends which can allow the chiropractor to play a pivotal role in managed care in the future."[56]

• Perhaps the single greatest contribution internationally has been made by the eminent British and Canadian orthopedic surgeon Professor William Kirkaldy-Willis. In the 1970s he began a clinical research collaboration with chiropractors at the Royal University Hospital, Saskatoon, at a time when this was contrary to his medical association's published ethic forbidding such a collaboration. He simply wrote advising his association of his plans and of the fact that he did not expect to hear any objection—his reputation was such that he did not.

Subsequently, through published research with chiropractic scientists— four editions of his widely acclaimed multidisciplinary text *Managing Low-Back Pain* which have featured chapters

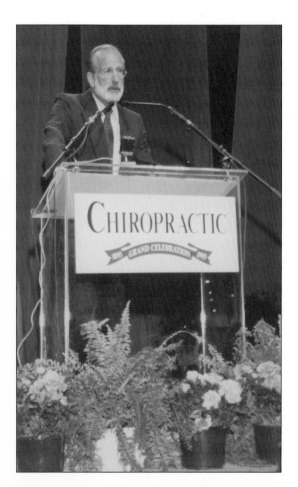

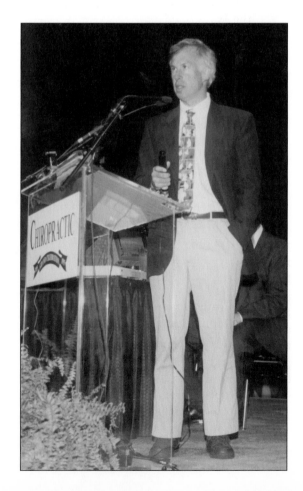

Orthopedic surgeons Dr. Arthur White, *left*, and Dr. Jim Weinstein, seen here speaking at the Chiropractic Centennial Foundation Conference at the Convention Center, Washington, DC, July 1995.

on manipulation by leading chiropractic researchers and himself, his work with Californian surgeon Dr. Aubrey Swartz in establishing the American Back Society which brought together all health disciplines managing patients with low-back pain, and otherwise—Kirkaldy-Willis has greatly advanced medical understanding and acceptance of the contribution the chiropractic profession can make to good patient care. In the preface to the second edition of *Managing Low-Back Pain* he wrote:

"Albert Einstein once said imagination is more important than knowledge, (and) there should be room in the physician's armamentarium for any type of knowledge and skill that will prove of value to the patient. We should be prepared to acknowledge new ideas from what H.R.H. The Prince of Wales calls *complementary medicine.*

"(I) believe that the physician of the future has much to learn by standing with feet firmly planted on the rock of orthodoxy in the low-back country, and reaching out to explore ideas that come from the borderland which separates orthodoxy from complementary practice. The interaction that occurs at this point produces the action."[57]

It is apparent from many sections of the present book, including the comments of Dr. Marc Micozzi which open this section on medical attitudes, that there is now broad medical acceptance of Kirkaldy-Willis' point of view. However few other physicians spoke so boldly of collaboration in the 1980s.

In this chapter we have seen that a substantial majority of the public, from all socio-economic groups, has had a positive attitude towards the acceptance and use of chiropractic services since the early 1980s. Now that the majority of physicians have similar attitudes, encouraged by further maturity in chiropractic education, research and practice during the past 10 years, it is clear that public attitudes will become even more positive.

References

1 Keating JC. BJ of Davenport: The Early Years of Chiropractic. Davenport, Iowa: Association for the History of Chiropractic, 1997:132.
2 Report of the committee of inquiry into chiropractic, osteopathy, homeopathy and naturopathy. Canberra, Australia: Australian Government Publishing Service, 1977.
3 Breen AC. Chiropractors and the treatmnent of back pain. Rheumatol Rehabil. 1977;16:46–53.
4 Wardwell WI. Chiropractic: history and evolution of a new profession, St Louis, Missouri: Mosby Yearbook, 1992. (See various studies quoted in Chapter 11, Acceptance of Chiropractic.)
5 Eisenberg DM, Kessler RC, et al. Unconventional medicine in the United States: prevalence, costs and patterns of use. New Engl J Med 1993;328:246–52.
6 Kelner M, Hall O, Coulter I. Chiropractors: do they help? Toronto, Ontario:Fitz-Henry and Whiteside, 1980.
7 Kelner M, Wellman B. Alternative health care? A profile of the users of five modes of treatment. J Alt Compl Med 1997;3:127–40.
8 Saunders Associates. The chiropractic profession. New York: The Public Relations Management Corporation, 1954. Quoted in Wardwell WI. Chiropractic: History and Evolution of a New Profession. St Louis, Missouri: Mosby Yearbook, 1992;231.
9 Gautvig M, Hvird A. Chiropractic in Denmark. Copenhagen, Denmark: Danish Pro-Chiropractic Association, 1975.
10 Astin JA. Why patients use alternative medicine: results of a national sStudy. JAMA 1998;279:1548–53.
11 Hurwitz EL, Coulter ID, et al. Use of chiropractic services from 1985 through 1991 in the United States and Canada, 1990-1997. JAMA 1998;280:1569–75.
12 Eisenberg DM, David RB, et al. Trends in alternative medicine use in the United States, 1990-1997. JAMA 1998;280:1569–75.
13 Ref 3 supra, 231
14 Millar WJ. Use of alternative health care practitioners by Canadians. Can J Pub Health 1997;155–158.
15 Carey TS, Garrett J, et al. The outcomes and costs of care for acute low-back pain among patients seen by primary care practitioners, chiropractors and orthopedic surgeons. New Engl J Med 1995;333:913–7.
16 The usage of and opinions about chiropractic services. Toronto, Ontario: Decima Research, Hill and Knowlton, 1998.
17 Stano M, Smith M. Chiropractic and medical costs for low-back care. Med Care 1996;34:191–204.
18 Sawyer CE, Kassak K. Patient satisfaction with chiropractic care. J Manip Physiol Ther 1993;16:25–32.
19 Ref 3 supra, 238.
20 Sanchez JE. A look in the mirror: a critical and exploratory study of public perceptions of the chiropractic profession in New Jersey. J Manip Physiol Ther 1991;14:165–76.
21 Sandhu DJ, Schoner B. Images of and attitudes toward B.C. health professionals. Vancouver, British Columbia: British Columbia Chiropractic Association, 1992.

22 Alternative medicine. Consumer 1997;366:20-7. (NZ Consumer Institute.)

23 Manga P, Angus D, et al. The effectiveness and cost-effectiveness of chiropractic management of low-back pain. Ontario, Canada: Pran Manga and Associates, University of Ottawa, 1993.

24 Manga P, Angus D. Enhanced chiropractic coverage under OHIP as a means of reducing health care costs, attaining better health outcomes and improving the public's access to cost-effective health services. Ontario, Canada: University of Ottawa, 1998.

25 Cherkin DC, McCornack FA. Patient evaluations of low-back pain care from family physicians and chiropractors. West J Med 1989;150:351–5.

26 Meade TW, Dyer S, et al. Low-back pain of mechanical origin: randomised comparison of chiropractic and hospital outpatient treatment. Br Med J 1990;300:1431–7.

27 Shekelle PG, Adams AH, et al. The appropriateness of spinal manipulation for low back pain: project overview and literature review. Santa Monica, California: RAND, 1991; Monograph No. R-4025/1–CCR/FCER.

28 Bigos S, Bowyer O, Braen G, et al. Acute low back problems in adults. Clinical practice guideline no. 14. Rockville, Maryland: Agency for Health Care Policy and Research, Public Health Service, U.S. Department of Health and Human Services, 1994.

29 Carlini WG, et al. Incidence of stroke following chiropractic manipulation. Proceedings of the American Heart Association's 19th International Joint Conference on Stroke and Cerebral Circulation. San Diego, California, 1994 and AHA news release.

30 Tettenborn B, et al. Postoperative brainstem and cerebellar infarct. Neurology 1993;43:471–7.

31 Cherkin DC, Deyo RA, et al. A comparison of physical therapy, chiropractic manipulation, and provision of an educational booklet for the treatment of patients with low-back pain. New Engl J Med 1998;339:1021–9.

32 The Des Moines Register, Iowa, October 8, 1998.

33 Chapman-Smith D, ed. Back pain, science, politics and money. The Chiropractic Report 1998; 12(6.)

34 Moore JS. Chiropractic in America. The history of a medical alternative. Baltimore, Maryland: Johns Hopkins University Press, 1993; Appendix B.

35 Ratti N, Pilling K. Back pain in the workplace. Br J Rheum 1997;36:260–4.

36 Jay TC, Jones SL, et al. A chiropractic service arrangement for musculoskeletal complaints in industry: a pilot study. Occup Med 1998;48:389–95.

37 Complementary medicine, new approaches to good practice. Oxford, England: Oxford University Press, British Medical Association, 1993.

38 MacLennan AH, Wilson DH, et al. Prevalence and cost of alternative medicine in Australia. Lancet 1996;347:569–73.

39 Use of alternative medicines and practices. Toronto, Ontario: Angus Reid, 1997.

40 An estimate based on an extrapolation of earlier figures in Ref 2 supra and Dickinson DPS. The growth of complementary therapy. Chapter 10. In: Ernst E, ed. Complementary medicine: an objective appraisal. Oxford, England: Butterworth-Heinemann, 1996.

41 Grenfel A, Patel N, et al. Complementary therapy: general practitioners' referral and patients' use in an urban multi-ethnic area. Comp Ther Med 1998;127–132.

42 Visser GJ, Peters C. Alternative medicine and general practitioners in the Netherlands: towards acceptance and integration. Fam Pract 1990;7:227–32.

43 Astin JA, et al. A review of the incorporation of complementary and alternative medicine by mainstream physicians. Arch Int Med 1998;158:2303–10.

44 Gordon NP, Sobel DS, et al. Use of and interest in alternative therapies among adult primary care clinicians and adult members in a large health maintenance organization. West J Med 1998;169:153–61.

45 Furnham A. Why do people choose and use complementary therapies? Chapter 5. In: Ernst E, ed. Complementary medicine: an objective appraisal. Oxford, England: Butterworth-Heinemann, 1996.

46 Robbins J. Reclaiming our health: exploding the medical myth and embracing the source of true healing. Tiburon, California: H.J. Kramer, 1996.

47 Jonas WB. Alternative medicine – learning from the past, examining the present, advancing to the future. JAMA 1998;280:1616–7.

48 Micozzi MS. Complementary care: when is it appropriate? Who will provide it? Ann Int Med 1998;129:65–6.

49 Report of the Ad Hoc Committee on Complementary Medicine, College of Physicians and Surgeons of Ontario, Toronto, adopted September 22, 1997.

50 Letter dated September 17, 1996 from the World Federation of Neurology (President) to the CIOMS (Secretary-General).

51 Patel-Christopher A. Family physicians and chiropractors: a need for better communication and cooperation. Toronto, Ontario: University of Toronto, 1990.

52 Aker P, Mior S, Hagino C. Utilization of chiropractic services in Ontario, Canada, unpublished abstract. Presented at the World Chiropractic Congress, London, England: World Federation of Chiropractic, 1993.

53 Coulter AH. A quest to integrate alternative medicine into conventional medicine: an interview with Woodson C. Merrell, MD. J Alt Comp Ther 1999;29–35.

54 Shekelle PG, Rogers WH, Newhouse JP. The effect of cost sharing on the use of chiropractic services. Med Care 1996;34:863–72.

55 Weinstein JN. Collaborative research. Conference Proceedings of the Chiropractic Centennial Foundation, Washington, DC: 1995;181.

56 White AH. Integration of chiropractic in managed care in a multidisciplinary setting. Conference Proceedings of the Chiropractic Centennial Foundation. Washington, DC: 1995;183–189.

57 Kirkaldy-Willis WH, ed. Managing low-back pain. 2nd Ed. New York: Churchill Livingstone, 1988.

CHAPTER 10

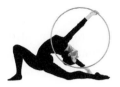

THE FUTURE OF CHIROPRACTIC

"Although chiropractic has arrived as an institutionalized part of America's health care system, arrival does not automatically confer permanent success . . . medical movements as well as individuals operate in a dynamic world of constant flux."

J. Stuart Moore, PhD, Historian, *Chiropractic in America, 1993.*[1]

A. Introduction

Health care systems in many countries are presently undergoing more rapid and dramatic change than ever before. A more informed public, seriously concerned about the lack of safety, ineffectiveness, impersonal nature and cost of much of mainstream health care, is increasingly taking control of health care decisions. There is the new integration of complementary and alternative medicine discussed in the previous chapter, with patients shopping for health. A true marketplace based on cost-effectiveness and patient satisfaction is eating into historical monopolies, and technology is providing sophisticated databases with score cards for individual patients and providers. A surplus of medical doctors, nurses and other health care providers is scavenging for a new scope of practice. What is the future of chiropractic in this evolving world?

This question was recently addressed in the U.S. in two expert reports from the Institute for Alternative Futures (IAF), a Washington, DC, institute which does health care forecasting in many countries and for the World Health Organization, and which was founded by prominent futurists Alvin Toffler and Clement Bezold. This chapter reviews the IAF reports, summarizes the most important internal and external factors that will influence the chiropractic profession's future and then makes several predictions.

B. The U.S.—Institute for Alternative Futures Reports

The two IAF reports, *The Future of Chiropractic: Optimizing Health Gains*[2] and *Future of Complementary and Alternative Approaches (CAAs) in U.S. Health Care*,[3] were commissioned by a leading U.S. chiropractic corporation that provides professional liability insurance and managed care services, the NCMIC Group.

NCMIC asked the IAF to look at the profession and U.S. health care trends and provide recommendations on what the profession needed to do in order to prosper over the next 10 years. The IAF's formal forecasting process included analysis of present facts and trends (based on its own database, consultation with leading practitioners and experts in health care generally and chiropractic, and focus groups with consumers, chiropractors and health care executives); identification of key factors; and then the development of several alternative scenarios or "plausible futures". Key points from the reports include:

1. In the next decade there will be an over-supply in all the major health care professions and fierce competition. Experts predict surpluses of 100,000 physicians and 200,000 nurses. There are 60,000 chiropractors in the U.S. today but, on current enrollments and predictions, that number will nearly double to 103,000 by 2010.

2. There will be much more public demand for complementary and alternative approaches

(CAAs) to health care including chiropractic/manipulation (currently the most used), oriental medicine/acupuncture, homeopathy, naturopathy, massage therapy and nutritional therapies. Successful primary medical care practices will have to include these CAAs.

3. Many physicians, nurses, physical therapists and others will try to learn and provide these CAAs themselves, but many others will work with specialists including chiropractors.

There are four possible scenarios for the U.S. chiropractic profession in 2010. On Scenario 1, chiropractors will be in Wal-Mart back centers and greatly increased demand will match increased supply

4. Success for all health professionals will be ruled by the quality of their data on results or—to use the technical term—outcomes. The key outcomes will be effectiveness, cost-effectiveness and patient satisfaction. To maintain and/or increase its market share the chiropractic profession must have convincing statistics from clinical practice with respect to specific health problems (e.g. headache, arthritis, asthma) and with respect to preventive/wellness care.

   Currently an estimated 14%–35% of chiropractic visits are for preventive/wellness visits but, even though the public will be demanding more services in this area, the role of chiropractors will be decreased unless they have the right supportive data. Reasons are that patients will also be looking to other CAAs, such as acupuncture and homeopathy, for preventive/wellness care, and greatly increased numbers of physicians, nurses and others will be seeking to provide CAAs themselves.

5. Managed care by 2010, contrary to what most people think, will not rebound from current cost management mistakes to return to something closer to the more familiar fee-for-service approaches. Managed care will dominate the marketplace but will be far more effective, prevention-oriented and customized. However one major source of managed care will be self-managed care—individuals and families, using the same information tools as managed care organizations, will choose to manage their own care privately, using only high-deductible catastrophic insurance as backup.

6. Three major priorities for the chiropractic profession are:

   • *To define its role in the rapidly changing health care system.* Are chiropractors spinal specialists, primary care providers, partners with medicine in mainstream health care or holistic practitioners alternative to and separate from the medical profession? The profession lacks a clear role in health care, and a serious coordinated effort from the grassroots up will be necessary to correct the problem. Without a clear and agreed upon role, and a shared vision, the profession will decline and suffer greatly in the near future because of new competitive pressures.

   • *To collect convincing data and practice statistics from clinical practice.* Currently this only exists for the management of patients with back pain, and to a lesser degree those with neck pain and headache. There must now be a similar effort in all significant areas of chiropractic practice.

   • *To develop the skills and capacities to work in many different health care environments.* Major changes lie ahead for everyone and the ability to be creative and integrate in various delivery systems is key to survival and growth.

7. There are four possible scenarios for the U.S. chiropractic profession in 2010. These are summarized in Table 1. On Scenario 1, the best for the profession and based on excellent new outcomes data proving chiropractic care is cost-effective for the conditions mentioned, chiropractors will be in Wal-Mart back centers and greatly increased demand will match increased supply.

   On Scenario 2, the worst and on which the profession has no shared vision or good data beyond low-back pain, the IAF sees little room for growth, a number of chiropractic colleges closing, and the proportion of spinal manipulation in the U.S. delivered by chiropractors dropping from 90% to 50%.

   In summary the IAF's reports are optimistic

Table 1 Overview of Four Scenarios for Chiropractic in 2010

Scenario 1—More and Better Health Care

Managed care, outcomes and consumers drive health care. Chiropractic care is proven cost-effective for low-back pain, headaches, neck pain, arthritis, scoliosis, asthma and repetitive stress injuries, and as supplementary therapy for cancer and other conditions where the disease or treatment involves significant pain. Wal-Mart creates "the back center" in its stores and expands access to low cost chiropractic care. There are 103,000 chiropractors, with average visits per week holding at about 120, with back conditions representing 50% of visits and wellness another 20%. Underemployment among chiropractors holds at about 15%.

Scenario 2—Hard Times, Frugal Health Care

Chiropractic is drastically affected by frugal universal coverage through managed care; outcomes limit manipulation to back problems. Meanwhile, 50% of spinal manipulation is delivered by physicians, nurses and other health professionals. Chiropractic colleges close, as only 68,000 chiropractors are needed in 2010. Many of those still practicing are forced to sell "the $10 treatment." Wellness visits decline and underemployment grows to 35%.

Scenario 3—Self-Care Rules

Very effective self-care, including advanced home health systems and universal catastrophic coverage, make health care a buyer's market. Individuals and families can do most of their care very effectively at home, lowering the need for all types of providers. Surplus providers exceed the 450,000 number forecast in the 1990s by the Pew Commission. Health care professionals who provide "touch" are in high demand but competition is fierce. Chiropractors are able to increase demand significantly by ensuring they provide care to 60% of those Americans with back problems (rather than 40% as in the 1990s.) Chiropractors also expand the indications they can treat with proven efficacy as well as provide evidence that for many people wellness visits are appropriate. The success of chiropractors leads to 85,000 chiropractors in 2010 (about 20,000 fewer than anticipated in 1997), but they are doing well.

Scenario 4—The Transformation

Chiropractors' clarified and expanded vision for the profession leads them to expand their contribution to health outcomes for their patients and their communities. Wellness and self-healing through enabling the body to function effectively (the innate healing force) becomes a much sought-after contribution of chiropractors through manipulation—so sought-after that 50% of manipulation in 2010 is performed by non-chiropractors. Chiropractors broaden what they do with and for their patients and their communities. For their patients they combine intelligent information systems with high touch and assertive coaching.

From Institute for Alternative Futures, 1998.[2]

---

if the chiropractic profession can adapt to the challenges of the era but sobering if it cannot. The future of chiropractic as a healing profession "will be shaped by a host of forces" but the greatest of these is "the identity and creativity of chiropractors . . . the future of chiropractic is in the hands of chiropractors themselves."

C. Internal and External Factors

The chiropractic profession has now established a permanent presence in the health care systems of many countries. The issue is whether that presence will expand or decline. What follows is a summary of the more important internal and external factors that will determine the degree of future success. Some of these are apparent from the IAF reports in the U.S., some not.

1. **Internal Factors**

   a) *A Clear and Agreed Identity and Role.* As long as chiropractic was a small profession only needing to attract under 10% of the population, and in circumstances where patients were free to make their own health care choices, there was no need for a clear identity. Because most practicing chiropractors have lived in such an environment until very recently —and in many countries still do—they have little appreciation of how much the lack of a clear identity is now hurting them.

   Do chiropractors offer mainstream primary care, a holistic alternative to primary medical care or specialist services in direct contact with the patient analogous to those of a dentist or optometrist? Are chiropractors prepared to work as part of a multidisciplinary team, including teams where the protocol provides a medical or nursing coordinator? These are questions about which the medical profession and the public remain unclear. As the historian Moore puts it, the current position is that chiropractors are "a somewhat curious mix of professional spine specialists still geared towards holistic systemic logic."[1] This mix is not necessarily bad—in fact it may be very good—but it is confusing, especially when most chiropractic organizations acknowledge an evolution to a specialized profession analogous to dentistry but others deny it.

In recent years there has been much greater agreement on the role of the profession by representative bodies such as the Association of Chiropractic Colleges and national chiropractic associations (see Chapter 5, pages 57–59). This role may be summarized as a primary contact profession specializing in the diagnosis, prevention and management of neuromusculoskeletal disorders by manual techniques, exercise, patient education and other natural methods. Practice settings range from individual private practice to multidisciplinary centers.

However there needs to be much greater acknowledgement and communication of this agreed identity. Quite simply, a product or service not understood is not used. The public and the medical profession need to appreciate:

- That chiropractic provides this specialized service, based on the fields of biomechanics, neurology and the manipulative arts, and addressing *functional* or movement pathology in the neuromusculoskeletal system rather than *structural* pathology;

- That there is no medical specialty that provides this service—which is why the chiropractic profession has grown and flourished; and

- The length and quality of the specialized education required—such an education, and the range of clinical skills it produces, cannot be achieved by other professions at an under-

graduate level or in part-time postgraduate courses.

b) *An International Identity*. This is of increasing importance in our global village. Some professions, such as osteopathy which is the equivalent of the medical profession in the U.S. but still has a scope of practice without drugs or surgery elsewhere, have lost this. Fortunately the chiropractic profession has internationally agreed standards of education and legal scope of practice, and maintenance of these will be essential to its continued growth and acceptance.

c) *Clinical and Research Outcomes Data Supporting the Profession's Agreed Role*. The importance of this point has already been addressed above (para 6, page 148), is understood by the profession's leadership and this should not provide an insurmountable challenge.

d) *Willingness and Ability to Adapt*. This is one of the hallmarks of success for any profession, business or enterprise in this era and perhaps poses the biggest challenge to the future of the chiropractic profession. This is because chiropractors, from their educational process right through to their leadership, must change from a posture of independence—often to the point of open criticism of other providers and their attitudes to health—to interdependence and teamwork. As Stephen Covey has explained in his *The 7 Habits of Highly Successful People*,[4] independence will get you some distance but wider success depends upon networking, teamwork, win-win solutions and interdependence.

Many individual chiropractors have these skills. There are also case examples from countries such as Denmark and Norway where the profession as a whole has re-positioned itself with the medical profession and health authorities. This starts with education. Most Danish and Norwegian chiropractic students are at Odense University where they share many common basic science classes with medical students during the first three years. Chiropractors and medical doctors leave a university setting where they both understand their complementary roles in the health care system. A 1998 publication by the Norwegian Chiropractic Association titled *An Introduction to Chiropractic Management: Disorders of the Neuromusculoskeletal System* and prepared for medical and other health providers is evidence-based, presents chiropractic as a neuromusculoskeletal specialty complementary to and respectful of medicine and physical therapy, and immediately led to much greater cooperation between the professions.[5]

There are similar trends in the U.K. and in Canada, where the two chiropractic colleges are now affiliated with York University in Toronto and the University of Quebec in Trois Rivières. But will the more volatile and divided chiropractic profession in the U.S. be willing and able to make this transition? In the U.S. chiropractic colleges remain private, independent, largely isolated from other health science faculties, and reliant upon alumni support.

2. **External Factors**

   a) *New competition in the field of spinal manipulation*. The single biggest external factor influencing the future of chiropractic—so new it is only now being recognized by the profession—is the recent arrival of competition in chiropractic's core field of skilled manual care for patients with musculoskeletal pain. Chiropractic has grown in a world where no other profession treated common back and neck pain confidently or well. Chiropractors could afford to be second or third choice with access and price disadvantages—enough patients would come to them in the end, find surprising relief after months of unsuccessful care, then tell their family and neighbors.

   The 1990s have finally seen the scientific and medical acceptance of spinal manipulation (see Section C in Chapter 8 and Chapter 7). At the same time clinical guidelines and peer leaders in medicine have rejected bedrest, most use of prescription drugs, most surgery and the physical therapy mainstays of passive machine therapies for most back pain patients. All of this represents a twin-edged sword for the chiropractic profession. It is now acknowledged that chiropractors have the correct approach, but

as a result other professions are seeking to duplicate their services.

Fortunately for chiropractors skilled assessment of joint and muscle function, the wide range of manipulative techniques necessary to relieve disorders in the young child, the adult male laborer of 250 lbs and the elderly lady with osteoporosis and arthritis, and the whole approach to patient management that arises from a chiropractic philosophy of health are not easily acquired by other providers. However current international experience suggests:

- On one hand there will be no major competition from medical doctors. Many will take short courses in spinal manipulation, meaning to practice this art, but few will persist. The great majority will simply appreciate the long education and full-time practice involved, and will end up referring more patients for skilled and specialist manual care. Those medical doctors who do practice will mostly practice part-time and at a rather crude skill level.

- However there is likely to be new competition from osteopaths, with British and French osteopaths bringing their traditional emphasis on manipulation back to North America and into other world regions. Additionally North American osteopathic schools will refocus on their manipulative roots as the over-supply of physicians provides a more competitive marketplace in general.

- There will also be significant competition from the physical therapy (PT) profession. PTs will not have the education and skill levels of chiropractors in biomechanics, manual assessment, treatment techniques and patient management, and unlike chiropractors they are not trained or licensed to diagnose, but many of their patients will get good results and never know the difference.

  PTs only learn rudimentary manual skills at undergraduate level, as part of a broad curriculum, and the majority practice in a variety of other areas such as hospital-based rehabilitation for cardiac patients, amputees and other post-surgical patients. However, initially in Scandinavia, Australia and New Zealand, and increasingly elsewhere, a significant number of PTs are doing formal postgraduate courses in manipulation. That branch of the profession is pushing for the right to direct patient contact and is changing from a predominantly female hospital-based workforce with part-time commitment to a mix of both men and women planning permanent careers in private enterprise rehabilitation practices. All the scientific evidence and clinical guidelines are pushing them towards rehabilitation based on manual treatments and exercise.

b) *Competition for access.* It is not sufficient to have excellent clinical skills if patients have little access to your services. The medical and nursing professions are in difficult times because of cost constraints, managed care and over-supply of graduates and organized medicine's containment of chiropractic—once done openly on supposed grounds of science and safety—is now focused at the level of access and economics.

No government in the world has required medical referral as a condition of chiropractic practice, knowing it was both unnecessary and would frustrate patient rights, but medicine has often been successful in establishing a gatekeeper function under private and public funding plans. Millions of Americans have been deprived of access to chiropractic services in the 1990s because of HMO medical gatekeepers.

In Canada, Denmark, Norway and Switzerland government plans fund chiropractic services chosen directly by the patient, but more recent funding arrangements in Italy and the U.K. rely upon medical referral for funding. Worker's compensation plans once all funded chiropractic services chosen by injured workers in the usual way—directly—but in New Zealand and some Australian states there is now a requirement of medical referral.

A major factor affecting the future of chiropractic in the next 10 years will be the ability of the profession through its associations and private networks of providers and entrepreneurs to maintain public/patient/union/employer support to the degree that there is success in legislative and contractual battles for direct patient access to funded chiropractic services. The battle will remain intense as competition increases.

D. A Few Predictions

1. *Chiropractic will accept a primary contact specialty role.* The profession will be forced to devote the majority of its energies to gathering clinical and other research data on, and expanding access to, its core market of manual care, exercise and education for the prevention and management of musculoskeletal pain. In this effort it will acknowledge its evolution to, and status as, a primary contact specialty:

   • In neuromusculoskeletal health (biomechanical problems in the locomotor system and their neurophysiological effects on health).

   • Utilizing natural methods, with a primary emphasis on manual care, exercise and patient education.

   Expressed as a scope of practice statement this specialty, which gives chiropractic a clear role in the health care system since there is no such medical practice, might be defined as:

   "The practice of chiropractic is the diagnosis, prevention and management of neuromusculoskeletal disorders through all methods of rehabilitation other than the use of prescription drugs and surgery, with a primary emphasis on manual treatments, exercise and patient education."

2. *Achievement of strong outcomes data and maintenance of leadership in spinal manipulation.* Aided by new government and public funding, and pushed by necessity, the profession will be successful in producing continued strong outcomes data showing that the results of chiropractic management of patients with the most common forms of musculoskeletal pain and headache are superior to other treatment approaches in terms of effectiveness, cost-

effectiveness and patient satisfaction. In the same way that chiropractic researchers have represented spinal manipulation on interdisciplinary guideline panels, written chapters on manipulation in interdisciplinary textbooks and are now on faculty at many medical schools and their teaching hospitals including even Harvard, chiropractors will retain their leadership in the art and science of manipulation.

3. *No expansion of scope of practice.* The profession will not seek the use of prescription drugs and surgery, and will not alter its undergraduate education to incorporate alternative forms of care such as acupuncture, naturopathy and homeopathy. Reasons include the fact that the increasing sophistication of the study of biomechanics, the relationship between mechanical disorders and altered neurophysiology, and specific manual techniques for different categories of patients will make these areas an evermore demanding full time field of education. There may be introductory courses on acupuncture and other disciplines, but education sufficient to form a basis for practice will be at a postgraduate level.

4. *Many physicians, nurses and physical therapists will re-qualify as chiropractors.* An increasing number of medical doctors, nurses and physical therapists will be given credits by chiropractic colleges and will re-qualify as chiropractors over a period of two to three years of study. This is already happening in several countries in Asia and Latin America and, as traditional barriers dissolve even further and medical doctors learn more of the quite sophisticated blend of manual skills and patient management skills in chiropractic education, many physicians determined to practice manipulation will seek the best education available. Ultimately, laws may one day force them to do so.

5. *Loss of market share and contraction of chiropractic education in North America.* Notwithstanding the above developments and the increased integration of chiropractic services, overall there will be an erosion of market share in North America as physicians, nurses, osteopaths and physical therapists develop education and practice in the field of manual care. Because many more musculoskeletal pain patients will receive manual care, chiropractors will see more patients

but their share will drop from over 90% to 50–60%. This means that U.S. chiropractic colleges must prepare for a period of some contraction. To counter smaller enrollments of North American students, several will enter distance education with campuses and/ or affiliations in other countries where there is an under-supply of chiropractors and the profession is in a period of strong growth. That path is already being followed by Palmer College in Brazil and the RMIT School of Chiropractic in Australia, Korea and Japan, and will become more common.

A related development in the U.S., following developments seen everywhere else in the chiropractic world, will be the affiliation of at least some chiropractic colleges with universities.

6. *Difficulties with identity and adaptation.* The loss of market share will be larger than it might have been, principally in the U.S., Canada and Australia, because of difficulties in developing a clear identity and role for chiropractors as providers of expert manual care of the neuromusculoskeletal system, complementary to medicine. These difficulties will arise because chiropractic colleges are too insular and resistant to change (a problem with all professions, but especially so where colleges are private and operate in isolation from other health sciences as with chiropractic education in the U.S.), because there is divided leadership and because the move from sturdy independence to integrated team health care will be too difficult for a significant number of chiropractors.

7. *Mergers are unlikely.* Ford has recently bought Volvo and Jaguar, and mega-mergers abound in our global marketplace. In theory there could be a breathtaking merger between chiropractic and osteopathy in the U.K., France and Australia, and an even more breathtaking international merger of chiropractic and that part of physical therapy/physiotherapy that now seeks to specialize in manual care. The fundamental reason would be to unite against the market power of the medical profession.

Chiropractic, osteopathy and latterly manipulative physical therapy are relatively small disciplines striving to maintain and/or gain independent access to patients legally and under third party payment systems. They could do much more together than apart, and united could probably force a halt to the inadequate, part-time short course postgraduate medical courses that are beginning to bring medical doctors into the field of spinal manipulation. However health care providers are professionals first and business people second, and such mergers are unlikely for various historical, attitudinal and professional reasons. There is no evidence anyone is even thinking about them.

E. Conclusion

1. Finally the future, perhaps 20 years distant yet, will see widespread recognition of the central concept of chiropractic health care that spinal functional disorders—the chiropractic subluxation—can mimic, aggravate or be a cause of many conditions apparently remote from the spine. Some infants with colic, some children with chronic recurring otitis media or asthma, some women with dysmenorrhea, some older adults with presumed cardiac pain, some senior citizens with chronic constipation, will be greatly relieved or "cured" by the diagnosis and treatment of spinal lesions that fall outside the current education and contemplation of physicians. Physicians and chiropractors must first build a bridge of trust on back pain and headache, but this will later lead to a wider path of understanding.

In all of the above cases the average family physician or medical specialist of 2020, working in a new interdisciplinary world combining medical and complementary care in a way not possible in the 20th century, will be aware that skilled biomechanical assessment and treatment of the spine may be an important option for many patients.

In the months prior to his death in September 1998, Dr. Virgil Strang, President of Palmer College, then in his 70s, reviewing his long life in chiropractic and the exciting developments of the past decade, stated more than once that he knew chiropractic principles and services would be fully accepted in the years ahead—the only question was whether they would be delivered by chiropractors or someone else.

As a fair-minded man with the interests of patients at heart he explained that, in the final analysis, he was unconcerned at the answer to this question. The chiropractic profession's mission had been to develop a discovery by D.D. Palmer in Davenport, Iowa in 1895 so that it was available to patients everywhere. As his life drew to a close he saw with pride that the ultimate success of that mission was assured. The following month Dr. N.V.K. Nair, Director, Health Infrastructure, Regional Office for the Western Pacific, World Health Organization, speaking at a symposium for chiropractic and medical doctors at De La Salle University, Manila, The Philippines—half a world distant from Davenport, Iowa—commented:

"Chiropractic is an accepted form of healing to the World Health Organization. Its acceptance, recognition and availability is gradually spreading in the countries of the Western Pacific.

"I am aware of the hesitation in so-called modern medical circles to accept chiropractic as their partners in lessening the suffering from specific conditions, especially musculoskeletal. Many forget the benefits of joining hands between modern and traditional medicine . . . Times have changed and now it is the customer's demand which is the crucial factor." [6]

The comments of Dr. Nair, a senior and respected health policy analyst from the Philippines, provide an apt point at which to close this book and enter a new era of improved health care—one in which patient interests of quality, effectiveness and cost take priority over the interests of health care professionals.

References

1   Moore JS. Chiropractic in America, 1993.
2   The future of chiropractic: optimizing health gains. Alexandria, Virginia: Institute for Alternative Futures, 1998.
3   Future of complementary and alternative approaches (CAAs) in U.S. health care. Alexandria, Virginia: Institute for Alternative Futures, 1998.
4   Covey SR. The 7 habits of highly effective people. New York: Simon & Schuster, 1989.
5   An introduction to chiropractic management: disorders of the neuromusculoskeletal system. Norwegian Chiropractors' Association, 1998.
6   Nair NVK. Address to a symposium on chiropractic in Asia, sponsored by De La Salle University and the World Federation of Chiropractic, De La Salle University, Manila, Philippines, October 2, 1998.

APPENDIX 1
ANATOMY OF THE NEUROMUSCULOSKELETAL SYSTEM: AN INTRODUCTION

The following pages illustrate the skeleton, the spine, the building blocks or basic structures of the spine, the back muscles, and the nervous system (central, peripheral and autonomic).

The Skeleton

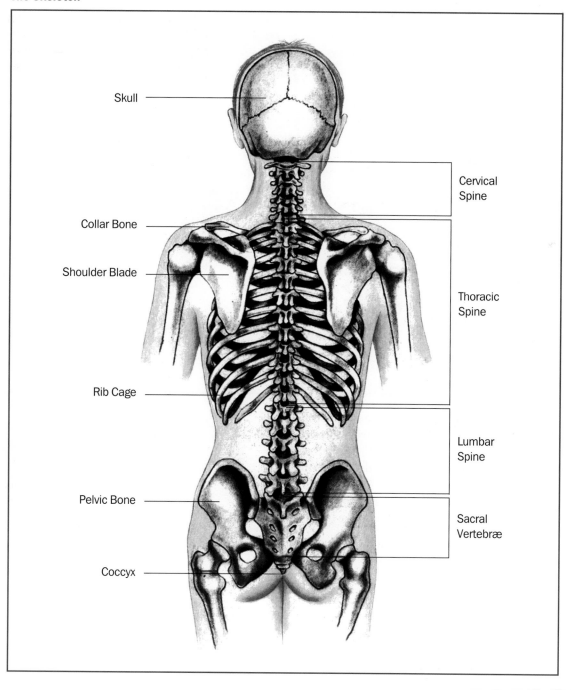

Skull

Cervical Spine

Collar Bone

Shoulder Blade

Thoracic Spine

Rib Cage

Lumbar Spine

Pelvic Bone

Sacral Vertebræ

Coccyx

The Structure of the Spine

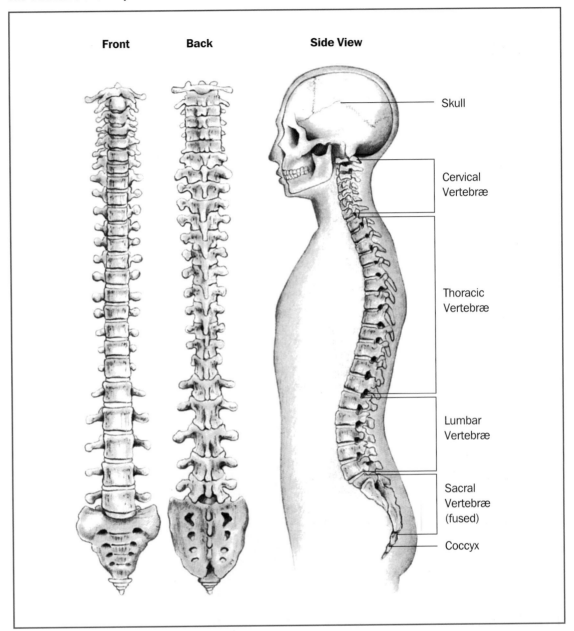

Front   Back   Side View

Skull

Cervical
Vertebræ

Thoracic
Vertebræ

Lumbar
Vertebræ

Sacral
Vertebræ
(fused)

Coccyx

Seen from the front or back, the normal spine should be straight, with no sideways curves. When viewed from the side, three distinct curves become visible: one inward curve in the neck (the cervical lordosis); one outward curve in the upper back (the thoracic kyphosis), and one inward curve in the lower back (the lumbar lordosis).

Building Blocks of the Spine

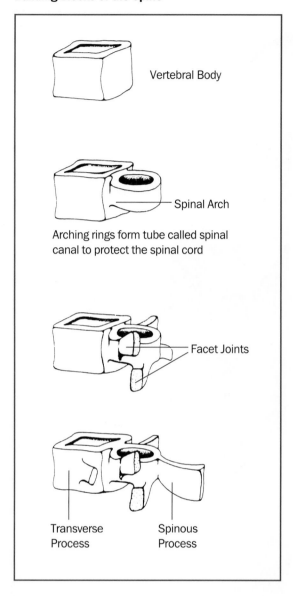

Vertebral Body

Spinal Arch

Arching rings form tube called spinal canal to protect the spinal cord

Facet Joints

Transverse Process

Spinous Process

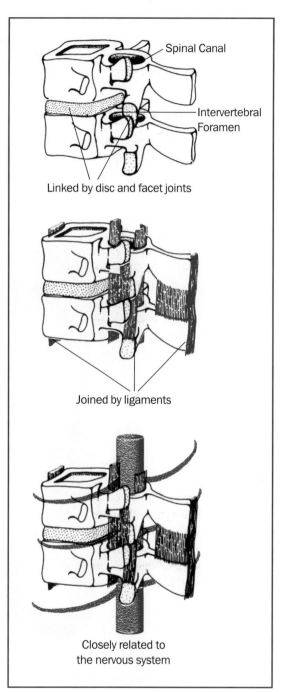

Spinal Canal

Intervertebral Foramen

Linked by disc and facet joints

Joined by ligaments

Closely related to the nervous system

These drawings illustrate the structure of a spinal vertebra, how it is linked to the vertebrae above and below, and the close relationship between the spine and the nervous system. The vertebrae are joined not only by ligaments (shown) but also by muscles, fascia and other connective tissue (not shown).

Between each pair of vertebrae two main spinal nerves exit from the central spinal cord through a passageway called the *intervertebral foramen* (IVF). These spinal nerves immediately form many branches that lead to all the spinal tissues (e.g. facet joints, disc, muscles, ligaments). Spinal nerves at one level (e.g. the space between the second and third lumbar vertebrae—known as L2-L3) have branches inner-

vating the spinal tissues not only at that joint level but also the levels above (L1-L2) and below (L3-L4). This is why the exact source of spinal pain in any given case can be such a diagnostic problem. Chiropractic motion palpation, specific movement of the joints and associated soft tissues to test for ranges of motion and movements that ease or provoke pain, is one diagnostic method that helps to isolate the source of pain.

The Muscles of the Back

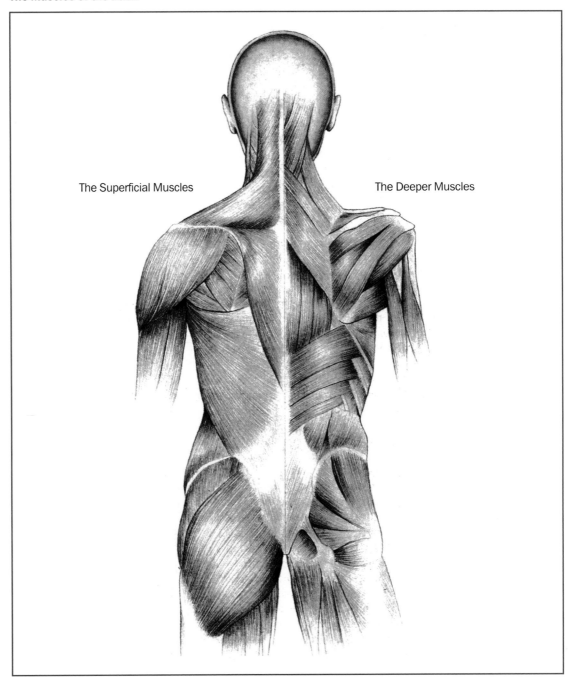

The Superficial Muscles   The Deeper Muscles

Many people think that the body is covered by a single layer of muscles. This is not the case, as can be seen if you look at the different layers of muscles on the back. Both a deep layer and a superficial layer of muscles cover the whole of the back area.

The Central Nervous System

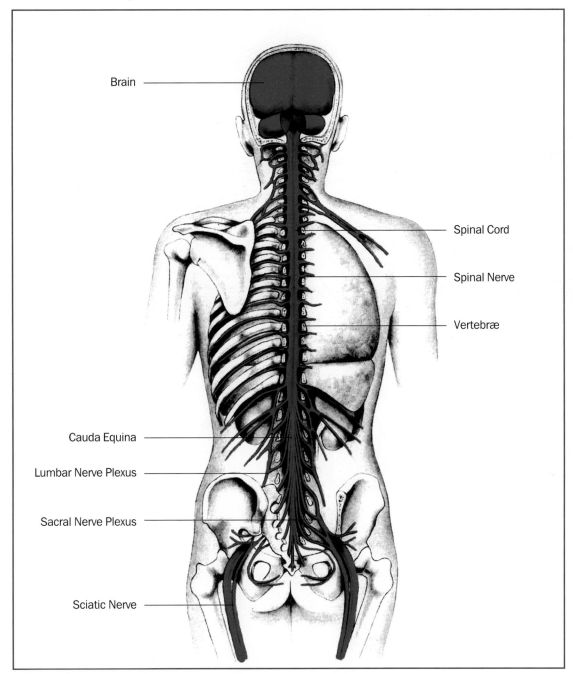

Brain

Spinal Cord

Spinal Nerve

Vertebræ

Cauda Equina

Lumbar Nerve Plexus

Sacral Nerve Plexus

Sciatic Nerve

The central nervous system consists of the brain, spinal cord and spinal nerves. The spinal cord arises from the base of the brain and passes down the spinal column. Arising from the spinal cord are the spinal nerves, which leave the spine between the vertebrae at each level to supply the various muscles, tissues and organs of the body.

The Peripheral Nervous System and the Autonomic Nervous System

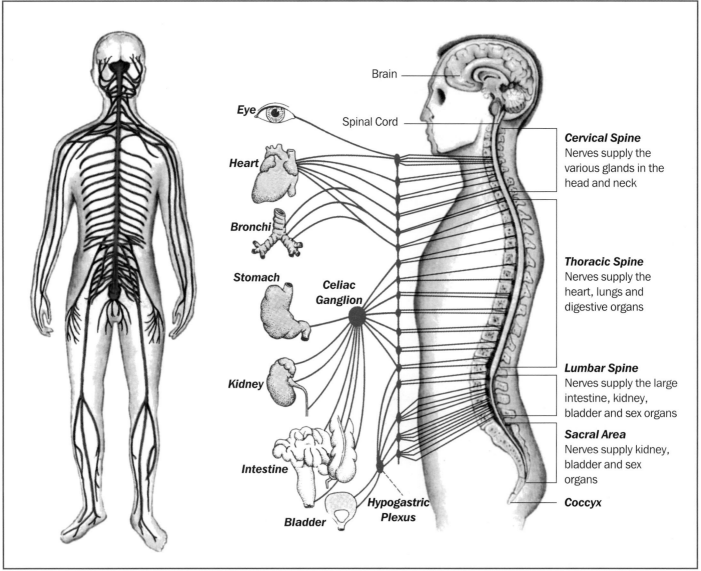

The peripheral nervous system starts from the spinal cord and nerves and passes to the periphery supplying the various parts of the arms, legs, chest and abdomen.

The autonomic nervous system supplies the various organs of the body. It is made up of the sympathetic and parasympathetic systems, which have opposite effects on the organs concerned.

APPENDIX 2
CREDITS FOR PHOTOGRAPHS AND FIGURES

Summary Facts on Chiropractic. *First photograph*: Courtesy David Byfield and Butterworth Heinemann (Byfield D, ed. Chiropractic manipulative skills, Oxford: Butterworth Heinemann, 1966.) *Second photograph*; Courtesy Ryan, Edwards and the Ontario Chiropractic Association.

Chapter 1. *Photograph on page 6*: Courtesy Sky City Photographers. *Photographs on page 10*: Courtesy Tom Bergmann.

Chapter 2. *Photograph on page 11*: Courtesy Robert Jackson and Palmer College of Chiropractic Archives. *Photographs 1 and 2 on page 13*: Courtesy Palmer College of Chiropractic Archives. *Photograph on page 14*: Courtesy Palmer College of Chiropractic Archives. *Photographs on page 17*: Courtesy Sky City Photographers. *Photographs on page 18*: Courtesy Gregory Cramer and Anton Rittling. *Photographs on page 20*: Courtesy World Federation of Chiropractic. *Photographs on page 22*: Courtesy Deborah Kopansky-Giles and Canadian Memorial Chiropractic College.

Chapter 3. *Illustrations on page 31*: Courtesy World Federation of Chiropractic. *Photographs on page 14*: Courtesy Carlan Stants.

Chapter 4. *Photographs on page 48*: Courtesy Japanese Association of Chiropractors and RMIT University School of Chiropractic, Tokyo. *Photographs on page 52*: Courtesy Jelloul Belhouari.

Chapter 5. *Photograph on page 62*: Courtesy British Chiropractic Association.

Chapter 6. *First two photographs on page 66*: Courtesy L. John Faye and the Motion Palpation Institute. *Photograph 3 and diagram on page 66*: Courtesy Tom Bergmann and Churchill Livingstone (Bergmann TF, Peterson DH, Lawrence DL, eds. Chiropractic technique. New York: Churchill Livingstone, 1993.) *Bottom left photograph on page 66*: Courtesy Susan Moore and Hamlyn Publishing (Moore S. Chiropractic: the art and science of body alignment. New York, NY: Harmony Books, 1989.) *Bottom right photograph on page 66*: Courtesy Hans Hadorn. *First two photographs on page 68*: Courtesy Palmer College of Chiropractic Archives. *Photograph 3 at left on page 68*:

Courtesy Tom Bergmann. *Photograph 4 at right on page 68*: Courtesy Carlan Stants. *Photograph 6 on page 68*: Courtesy Craig Liebenson. *Photographs on page 70*: Courtesy Tom Bergmann. *Photograph on page 76*: Courtesy Ryan, Edwards and the Ontario Chiropractic Association. *Photographs on page 79*: Courtesy Claudia Anrig and Gregory Plaugher. *Photographs on page 88*: Courtesy Susan Moore and Hamlyn Publishing (Moore S. Chiropractic: the art and science of body alignment. New York, NY: Harmony Books, 1989.)

Chapter 7. *Figure 1 on page 99 and Figure 2 on pages 100-101*: Courtesy David Cassidy and Churchill Livingstone (Kirkaldy-Willis WH, Bernard TN, eds. Managing low-back pain. 4th ed. New York: Churchill Livingstone, 1999.)

Chapter 8. *Photograph on page 109*: Courtesy World Federation of Chiropractic. *Photographs and figures on page 114*: Courtesy Tom Bergmann and Churchill Livingstone (Bergmann TF, Peterson DH, Lawrence DL, eds. Chiropractic technique. New York: Churchill Livingstone, 1993.) *Figure 3 on page 117*: Courtesy David Imrie, Lu Barbuto and Stoddart Publishing (Imrie D, Barbuto L. The back power program. Toronto, Ontario: Stoddart Publishing, 1988.)

Chapter 9. *Photographs on page 126*: Courtesy Chiropractic Centennial Foundation and World Federation of Chiropractic. *Illustrations on page 131*: Courtesy World Federation of Chiropractic. *Photographs on page 139*: Courtesy Marion MacGregor and John Triano. *Photographs on page 140*: Courtesy Bill Defoyd. *Photographs on page 142*: Courtesy Peter DeFranco, Shelby Elliott and Louis Sportelli. *Photographs on page 144*: Courtesy World Federation of Chiropractic.

Appendix 1. *Anatomical drawings on page 157, 158, 160, 161 and 162*: Courtesy Susan Moore and Hamlyn Publishing (Moore S. Chiropractic: the art and science of body alignment. New York, NY: Harmony Books, 1989.) *Anatomical drawings on page 159*: Courtesy David Imrie, Lu Barbuto and Stoddart Publishing (Imrie D, Barbuto L. The back power program. Toronto, Ontario: Stoddart Publishing, 1988.)

About the Author

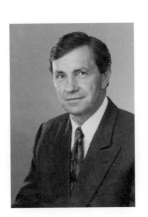

Mr. David Chapman-Smith received his honors degree in law from Auckland University, New Zealand in 1972 and was a litigation partner in the firm of Holmden Horrocks & Co. in Auckland until his emigration to Canada in 1982. He was then admitted to the bar in Ontario where he practises in Toronto.

His introduction to chiropractic was as counsel for the New Zealand Chiropractors' Association before the New Zealand Commission of Inquiry into Chiropractic in 1979. He currently acts as Secretary-General for the World Federation of Chiropractic and General Counsel for the Ontario Chiropractic Association. He is a former member of the Board of Advisors of the American Back Society.

Mr. Chapman-Smith, who is the author of many articles in the medico-legal and chiropractic literature, is a co-editor of national chiropractic clinical guidelines in each of the United States and Canada, and for the past 13 years has been editor of a newsletter titled *The Chiropractic Report* (www.chiropracticreport.com).

His wife holds dual qualifications in medicine and chiropractic, and two of his brothers are physicians.